THE DIRT

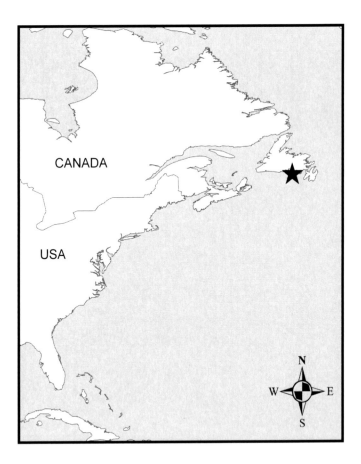

CANADA

USA

N
W E
S

THE DIRT

Industrial Disease and Conflict
at St Lawrence, Newfoundland

Rick Rennie

Fernwood Publishing • Halifax & Winnipeg

Editing: Judith Kerans and Brian Turner
Cover design: John van der Woude
Cover art: Detail from a mural painted by Boyd Holloway,
used courtesy of the St. Lawrence Heritage Society
All photographs courtesy of and used by permission from St. Lawrence Memorial Miners'
Museum; courtesy of the Town Council of St. Lawrence, Newfoundland.
Printed and bound in Canada by Hignell Book Printing

Published in Canada by Fernwood Publishing
Site 2A, Box 5, 32 Oceanvista Lane
Black Point, Nova Scotia, B0J 1B0
and #8 - 222 Osborne St., Winnipeg, Manitoba, R3L 1Z3
www.fernwoodpublishing.ca

This book has been published with the help of a grant from the Canadian Federation for the
Humanities and Social Sciences, through the Aid to Scholarly Publications Programme, using
funds provided by the Social Sciences and Humanities Research Council of Canada.

Fernwood Publishing Company Limited gratefully acknowledges the financial support
of the Government of Canada through the Book Publishing Industry Development
Program (BPDIP), the Canada Council for the Arts and the Nova Scotia
Department of Tourism and Culture for our publishing program.

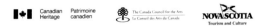

Library and Archives Canada Cataloguing in Publication

Rennie, Rick, 1962-
The dirt: industrial disease and conflict at St. Lawrence, Newfoundland / Rick Rennie.

Includes bibliographical references.
ISBN 978-1-55266-259-5

1. Fluorspar industryHealth aspects—Newfoundland and Labrador—St. Lawrence. 2. Fluorspar
industry—Employees—Diseases—Newfoundland and Labrador—St. Lawrence. 3. Fluorspar
industry—Employees—Health and hygiene—Newfoundland and Labrador—St. Lawrence. 4.
Miners—Health and hygiene—Newfoundland and Labrador—St. Lawrence. 5. Mineral dusts—
Toxicology—Newfoundland and Labrador—St. Lawrence.I. Title.

HD7269.M61C36 2008   363.17'99   C2007-906985-1

CONTENTS

To the memory of my parents, Albert J. Rennie and Mary B. Rennie

ACKNOWLEDGEMENTS

The author thanks the following organizations and individuals:

the Institute of Social and Economic Research, Memorial University, the J.R. Smallwood Centre for Newfoundland Studies, Memorial University, and the Social Sciences and Humanities Research Council of Canada for their financial support of this research; the Town Council of St. Lawrence for access to archival sources; Lawrence Issac for his cartography work; Herbert Slaney, Jerome Spearns, Richard (Bud) Loder, the late Adrian Slaney, the late Richard Clarke, Jerome Slaney, Shannon Ryan, Allan Seager, Beth Oberholtzer, Gregory Quirke, Wayde Rowsell and Barbara Neis; Gregory Kealey for his assistance and advice over the years; Marianne, Charlie and Joseph Rennie; and Ingrid Botting, a true friend and a constant source of guidance and support.

the folks at Fernwood Publishing — Beverley Rach, Debbie Mathers, Brenda Conroy, and Wayne Antony; to Brian Turner and Judith Kearns for copy editing the manuscript; to three anonymous reviewers who provided useful suggestions for revising the manuscript.

This book has been published with the help of a grant from the Canadian Federation for the Humanities and Social Sciences, through the Aid to Scholarly Publications Programme, using funds provided by the Social Sciences and Humanities Research Council of Canada.

INTRODUCTION

In 1933, in the midst of the Great Depression, a group of men at St. Lawrence on the south coast of Newfoundland hauled some rundown mining equipment over the barrens and swamps and started hacking out the fluorspar buried in the granite hills west of town. During subsequent decades, mining became an industry in the region, expanding to include a number of mines and processing facilities run by American and Canadian-based employers, and providing steady employment for hundreds from St. Lawrence and neighbouring communities. But a heavy price was extracted in exchange: by the time the last mine was shut down, fifty years later, some two hundred workers had been killed by silicosis, cancer, and other illnesses caused by the dust and radiation that permeated the mines.

Growing up a couple of miles from St. Lawrence, attending school and doing much of my socializing there, I was, like others, keenly aware that a tragedy had taken place and was continuing to unfold before our eyes. It was a fairly common experience to trek from school to church for the funeral of some child's father. Many homes held men whose bodies had been ravaged by disease or widows left with meagre support to raise their children. The talk was sprinkled with references to "the dirt" — the general name given to multiple miners' diseases — to who had or hadn't been approved for workers' compensation benefits, or to how long a particular person might have to live.

Those outside the St. Lawrence area who are aware of the disaster have likely learned of it through Elliot Leyton's 1975 book *Dying Hard*. Based on a series of interviews with ailing miners and with women in the community, *Dying Hard* revealed much about the physical, social, psychological, economic, and other effects of industrial disease and about people's experience with the workers' compensation system. *Dying Hard* accomplished its goal of drawing attention to the St. Lawrence situation, and I see that book not only as instrumental in revealing important aspects of the St. Lawrence story but also as an important *part* of that story, as will become apparent. My book differs from Leyton's in that it explores the many economic, social, political, and other forces that created the St. Lawrence disaster and the response to it. The state of local medical facilities, rivalry among union leaders, technological changes, the media, Quebec separatism, wars, and national and provincial politics are just a few of the many diverse factors encompassed by this analysis.

Among the several themes running through this chronicle, none emerges as more compelling than the persistent efforts by workers, the union, community activists, and others to achieve recognition of workplace hazards and the diseases they produced, to have those hazards addressed, and to obtain adequate support for victims and their families. As noted by Alan Derickson, perhaps the foremost American historian working in the area of occupational health and industrial disease, the widespread view that sees those killed and incapacitated by industrial disease as simply victims of forces entirely beyond their comprehension and influence is rooted largely in our lack of understanding about past struggles by workers and others around workplace hazards and their effects (1988b, xii–xiii). One advantage of my approach is that it not only considers the issues of exploitation and victimization but also provides for going beyond that to incorporate the themes of struggle and conflict. In short, it allows for seeing those affected by the disaster as victims, which they surely were, but not as passive and unknowing, for in many ways they acted on their knowledge and beliefs to try to improve their situation. This approach also underscores that those in such situations are victims not just of the immediate hazards to which they are exposed but of the economic, political, social, and other forces that work — deliberately or otherwise — to stifle their claims and restrict their ability to take effective action.

As an account of the many layers and dimensions of the St. Lawrence disaster, this book is framed by a number of theoretical considerations. These include the classic "jobs or health" dilemma in which workers so often find themselves, especially in contexts where employment alternatives are limited. In such situations, workers often aim to preserve both their health and their jobs, and thus to seek a balance between exerting sufficient pressure to have their concerns addressed and avoiding the loss of the industry and their jobs (cf., Storey and Lewchuk 2000). Novek describes this process as going beyond the simple "wages for effort" bargain to a "wages for effort and health" bargain, which includes an aspect of workers determining whether or not the actual or potential effects on their health are acceptable in exchange for wages and jobs (1992, 18). Workers' ability to manage this tension effectively is in turn influenced by a number of considerations, including the demand for their labour and the ability of an employer to acquire the industry's product elsewhere, factors that constantly change over time. In this light it is not surprising that a long-term study of the American coal mining industry concluded that the business climate was the key determinant in shaping struggles around health and safety (Wallace 1987), or that a survey of industrial fatalities in Canada over the twentieth century reached a similar conclusion, noting that economic conditions were an overriding influence (Suschnigg 1989).

The issue of workers establishing an acceptable situation within the "jobs or health" dilemma is key in addressing the common question of why workers engage at all in work they know to be damaging or potentially damaging to their health. From the perspective of the classical economist, this question is best answered in the context of market forces: workers engage in such occupations in exchange for what they consider to be appropriate offsetting compensation, such as "danger pay," and in the absence of such compensation will seek employment elsewhere (Dorman 1996, 26–31). In addition to assuming that workers actually have knowledge of the hazards to which they are exposed, and ignoring that many of the world's most dangerous jobs are also among the lowest paying, this view fails to consider that workers may be strongly tied to even dangerous jobs through the limits imposed by their education and skills, as well as by strong personal, social, and cultural reasons for wanting to stay in a particular location (Derickson 1988b, 75–76).

Where labour relations is the arena in which much of the conflict and struggle regarding health hazards takes place, it is important to consider the relationship between occupational health and safety and labour relations. Bargaining power, legal protections, and access to information and support are just some of the positive influences that unionization and the formal labour relations system can have in helping workers address occupational hazards. However, the labour relations system that has dominated industrialized countries over the past half-century or so (often called the "Fordist" model), may also have drawbacks in this regard. For example, the system's strict rules regarding why and when a work stoppage is legitimate may not be well suited to dealing with hazards that arise or are recognized in sudden and unpredictable ways (Beaumont 1983, 49–51; Gunderson and Swinton 1981, 5.7–5.8). The size and structure of the organization representing workers are also important considerations. Affiliation with a large organization can empower a smaller, local union in many respects but can also result in a lack of attention to the health concerns in a particular workplace (Bacow 1981, 98–99). Another important consideration is how the industrial relations system interacts with health and safety legislation. Sometimes, the simple existence of protective legislation can serve as a rationale for not dealing with health and safety concerns within the labour relations arena. However, when legislation exists but is not enforced it may actually erode a union's ability to make progress. In addition, health and safety laws are necessarily generic because they must be applicable to a vast range of industries and situations. However, hazards are usually specific to a given workplace and work practices and require specific, targeted measures (Sass 1979, 75).

These dynamics likely contribute to the fact that health and safety struggles are often carried out through informal channels such as union and citizen lobbying, wildcat strikes, and other forms of protest rather than in the more formal arenas of contract negotiations and authorized strikes. In addition, it appears that while grievances over health and safety may not be the official, explicit issue at stake in job actions, they are often an underlying cause of labour unrest (Ison 1979; Reasons et al. 1981).

Employers as well as workers confront a range of sometimes conflicting demands when it comes to occupational health concerns. Central among these is the relationship between generating profits and protecting the work-force. Novek describes this relationship as rooted in the fact that "a satisfactory level of occupational health is necessary to maintain productivity in an industrial society and yet resources devoted to workplace health and safety can detract from profitability" (1992, 17). One way of viewing this matter is through Marx's concept of the reproduction of labour power, as summarized in his statement that if a worker works today, "tomorrow he must again be able to repeat the same process in the same conditions as regards health and strength" (Marx 1977, 168). While Marx is referring primarily to the fact that workers must be provided with at least the basic means of physical subsistence (such as food and shelter) if they are to reproduce their labour power, the concept can readily be applied to protecting workers' health and safety at a level that will allow for further extraction of labour power. Furthermore, it is often not enough simply to preserve the health of a workforce so that it is able to reproduce its labour power; it is also necessary to address workers' fears and grievances about health hazards. While a disabled workforce *cannot* provide the labour necessary for profitable production, a mistrustful and hostile one *will not* do so.

The extent to which employers will go in preserving an able and willing workforce is determined by a number of factors. The labour supply plays a significant role, as employers will be less concerned with addressing grievances when workers are more easily replaced. There is also the possibility of shifting production elsewhere to reduce the costs of maintaining an adequately healthy and/or compliant workforce. An employer may also use the threat of shifting production as a way of stifling unrest.

In addition to the possibility of creating an unproductive workforce, employers must also consider other liabilities that might result from not addressing health hazards, including those associated with workers' compensation. Ideally, workers' compensation not only provides financial and other support in cases of disability but also motivates employers to maintain safe and healthy workplaces by linking premium levels to claims, much like other forms of insurance. However, a number of factors influence how well the system performs this function, including whether individual employers are actually held liable for claims arising from their operations and whether certain illnesses are covered under workers' compensation.

The issue of workers' compensation coverage can be especially problematic when it comes to industrial disease. Unlike injuries, which can usually be linked to an identifiable source, the connection between working conditions and illnesses is often unclear because of such factors as inadequate understanding of hazards, the time lapse between exposure and illness, and the existence of multiple ailments (Burke 1985; Derickson 1988a). Furthermore, much of our knowledge about the incidence of industrial disease comes from data complied by workers' compensation boards, data that often includes only those workers covered by workers' compensation (currently about 80 percent across Canada), only those conditions that are covered, and often only those claims that are accepted (Müller 1985, 134). It has been argued therefore that such statistics may conceal more than they reveal and that they often represent "only the tip of the submerged mass of illness" (Weindling 1985, 11). Such factors often create disagreement over the number and types of illnesses deemed to be work-related or to be worthy of compensation coverage, resulting in what Bayer describes as the polarization between the "minimalist" and the "maximalist" positions, with the former characterized by attempts to limit as much as possible the recognition of diseases as work-related and the latter by attempts to extend that recognition as far as possible (1988, 7).

The characteristics of industrial disease can also affect the emergence of awareness about the nature, extent, and even the existence of a disaster. When a number of workers die in a single workplace accident, there is usually little question that a disaster has occurred or about the scope of that disaster (Tucker 2006). Such events also tend to draw considerable public and media attention, partly because there is a dramatic occurrence and a single location upon which to focus that attention. However, when even a considerable number of workers die individually over a period of time, as they do from industrial disease, it tends to provoke little public outrage or attention (Baldwin 1977). Learning about a disaster involving industrial disease, moreover, can be a longer and more protracted process. It can also be far more than a medical or scientific matter, because the way that knowledge is gathered, suppressed, spread, and manipulated is shaped by a host of medical, social, economic, political, and demographic factors (Graebner 1988).

The fact that disasters involving industrial disease tend to attract relatively little public attention, along with the diverse theoretical and thematic concerns involved, may help explain why the subject area of this book has been largely neglected by historians in Canada. While the historical literature on mining and miners' unions contains references to such matters as occupational hazards and workers' struggles regarding them, there is little in the way of detailed analysis. Moreover, the historical accounts of industrial disasters that do exist focus almost exclusively on safety rather than health hazards, and on injuries (usually involving multiple fatalities) rather than industrial diseases (David 1976; Bercuson 1978; McKay 1984; Lunn and Palmer 1997; McCormick 1992). The same is true of Great Britain, where the vast majority of the literature deals with the institutional and political dimensions of miners' unions or with the culture of mining and mining communities (a notable exception being Paul Weindling's 1985 collection on the social history of occupational health). The literature is far more developed in the United States, where several key works have added greatly to our knowledge of the history of health hazards and industrial disease in the American mining industry, including Alan Derickson (1988b and 1998a), David Rosner and Gerald Markowitz (1987), and David Rosner (1992). Others who have contributed important studies dealing with health hazards and industrial diseases in mining and other contexts in the United States are Collis and Greenwood (1977), Wedeen (1984), Robinson (1991), Caulfield (1989), Judkins (1986), Smith (1987), and Bartrip (2006).

The role of the government is also crucial in understanding the recognition of and response to occupational hazards. For example, because of its role in such areas as the workers' compensation system and the medical system, government can play an important part in the process of determining the nature and extent of work-related diseases. However, the attitudes and actions of government in this respect are influenced by a number of considerations. For example, determining the true extent of work-related illnesses might lead to liabilities for employers or other results that threaten industries and jobs. The same considerations can affect the government's willingness to impose fines or take other actions to force employers to comply with health and safety legislation. Such factors underscore the political economy dimensions of health hazards and industrial disease in an industry such as mining. Given that it generally involves an outlay of capital and technology that can be provided only by large private interests, the mining industry is a common context for a relationship of dependence to emerge. This explains why mining is a frequent theme in much of the literature on foreign dependence and its associated ills (Gjording 1991; Lanning and Mueller 1979; O'Faircheallaigh 1984; Cunningham 1981; Daniel 1979). In Newfoundland, dependence on foreign developers has long been a heavy influence on the actions of successive governments in their attempts to diversify the economy and provide jobs in a situation of chronic unemployment (Alexander 1974; 1976a; 1978; Antler 1979; Reeves 1989; Summers 1994), and this was consistently an overriding factor in the state's response to the St. Lawrence situation.

An overriding theme that draws together many of the trends and topics addressed here is the process of "externalization." In this context, externalization refers to the practice of employers off-loading the costs of production, including the cost of health impacts, onto workers, their families, governments, and other parties. Simply put, in a given situation an employer may "internalize" costs by investing in measures that will reduce workplace hazards and/or by paying the cost of illnesses arising from those hazards.

However, what employers often seek to do is have someone else bear those costs, and the element of dependence that marks the relationship of both workers and governments to employers contributes to this process (Quinlan 1999; Dorman 2000, Rosenstock et al. 2005).

I have made use of a wide range of sources in this book. In addition to the secondary literature on occupational health and safety, labour history, industrial relations, workers' compensation, and other related topics, this study draws on archival materials, newspapers, government documents, and oral interviews. The key archival sources include a sizeable collection of union and other documents held at the St. Lawrence Memorial Miners' Museum, spanning the period from the early 1940s to the late 1970s. The Provincial Archives of Newfoundland and Labrador were also a valuable source, particularly the records of the Commission of Government (GN 38), the Newfoundland and Labrador Department of Health (GN 78), and the Royal Commission Respecting Radiation, Compensation and Safety at the Fluorspar Mines, St. Lawrence, Newfoundland (GN 6). The archives of the Aluminum Company of Canada in Montreal supplied some information on that company's operations, though the records provided to me contained almost nothing on health and safety or labour relations. The Confederation of National Trade Unions in Quebec apparently has an archival collection that might have proved useful, but was uncooperative when approached.

Oral interviews are also a key source. The Memorial University of Newfoundland Folklore and Language Archive (MUNFLA) holds a number of interviews conducted in the 1960s with Newfoundland labour leaders, including three presidents of the miners' union at St. Lawrence. In addition, I conducted interviews with several former miners at St. Lawrence, which were especially useful as first-hand accounts of early suspicions among workers and others about the relationship between the working environment and illnesses among miners, as a counter-balance to official descriptions of working conditions, and as a source of information and opinions on episodes of labour and social unrest. One of the sad facts of doing oral history on an industrial disaster is that many of those affected are not alive to tell their stories. The selection of informants is based partly on this fact and partly on seeking to speak with individuals who worked in the mines at different periods across a broad span of time.

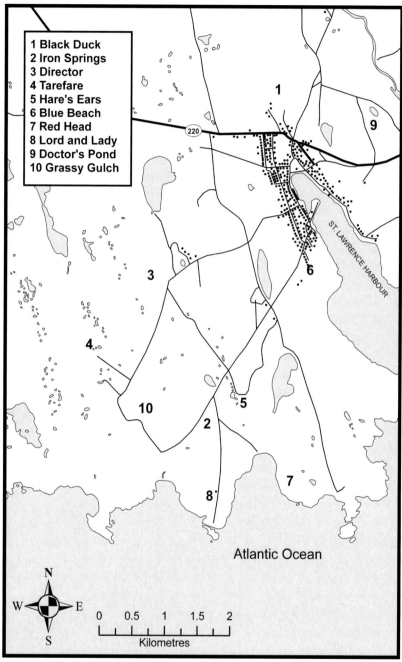

1 Black Duck
2 Iron Springs
3 Director
4 Tarefare
5 Hare's Ears
6 Blue Beach
7 Red Head
8 Lord and Lady
9 Doctor's Pond
10 Grassy Gulch

Atlantic Ocean

ST. LAWRENCE HARBOUR

220

Location of Mine Sites in Relation to the Community

Chapter One

ORIGINS OF A DISASTER
Working Conditions and Labour Relations in the 1930s

The Historical Background

Like hundreds of other towns around the coast of Newfoundland, St. Lawrence originally served as a base for the migratory cod fishery. Basque fishermen were operating out of the town as early as the sixteenth century, before being displaced by the English and Irish who eventually settled the area. By the early 1900s, St. Lawrence, its economic base the production of salt cod for foreign markets, was home to about 800 people. The fishery was carried out primarily by small crews, often family-based and governed by a system under which local merchants advanced goods that were paid for with cured fish at the end of the season. Producers were almost perpetually in debt and rarely saw cash.

By the 1920s, international competition and other factors had led to a decline in the Newfoundland cod fishery. By 1930 the fishery could no longer provide a livelihood for many and a large portion of the population was dependent on public relief (Alexander 1976a, 229–48; Summers 1994, 92–97; Neary 1988, 12–43). For Newfoundland, therefore, the onset of the Great Depression was the nadir of an ongoing decline.

The virtual collapse of the island's main industry had serious consequences for many communities, but in the St. Lawrence area, the economic crisis was exacerbated by a natural disaster. On November 18, 1929, the region was struck by a tidal wave originating from an undersea earthquake approximately 200 miles to the south. A massive wave and high tides devastated communities along the east side of the peninsula, claiming twenty-seven lives and sweeping away houses, fishing facilities, boats, and supplies. There was no loss of life in St. Lawrence but more than thirty boats were lost or destroyed and many buildings and their contents swept out to sea. The people of St. Lawrence were described as "dazed and destitute" (*Daily News* November 23, 1929, 3), and a government inspector described the scene there as one of "desolation," with the people "in a state of dire destitution" (Newfoundland 1929). In addition to the other damage, the tidal wave appears to have added to the problems in the fishery. One resident recalled that "for many years afterwards the codfish and bait failed to come to our shores" (Slaney 1975, 2), while another observed that the fishery "has been practically a failure every year since the tidal wave."[1]

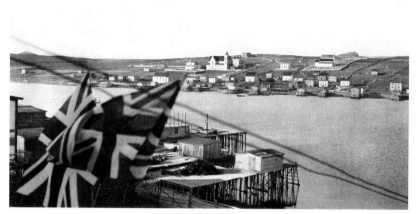

View of the east side of St. Lawrence, c. 1937. The large building in the centre is the Roman Catholic church and the smaller one to the right the Anglican church. Note also the Union Jack in the foreground, a symbol of historical connection to Britain.

Under these circumstances, it is not surprising that a New York entrepreneur found willing participants when he proposed in 1932 to establish an industry to mine and export the fluorspar deposits in the area. "Fluorspar" is a popular commercial name for a non-metallic mineral composed of calcium and fluoride (its chemical formula is CaF_2). It usually occurs as veins within the crevices of surrounding rock such as granite or limestone. It has a number of commercial uses, depending on the proportion of CaF_2 to other ingredients in the ore. The three basic grades are "acid," which is used

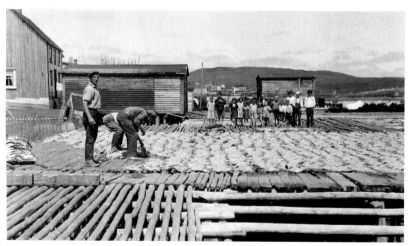

The pre-mining economy: drying salt cod at St. Lawrence, c. 1937.

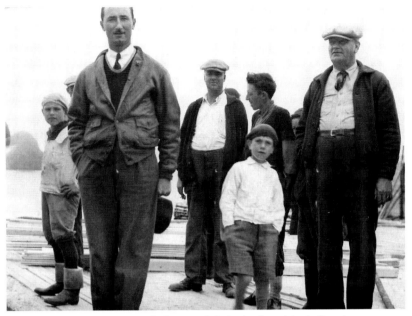

Walter Seibert (left foreground) on a St. Lawrence dock shortly after arriving by float plane.

in making hydrofluoric acid for, among other things, smelting aluminium; "ceramic," which is used in making glass and ceramics; and "metallurgical," which is used primarily in making steel. Fluorspar must usually be refined to varying degrees to make it useful for these purposes.

At the time this proposal was put to the people of St. Lawrence, fluorspar had been mined in various parts of the world for about fifty years. The major American sites were in Illinois and Kentucky, while in Canada fluorspar had been mined near Madoc, Ontario, from 1916 to 1920. The American mines were substantial operations, producing up to 80,000 tons a year, while the Madoc mines produced considerably less (Fellman 1926, 197–211).

The St. Lawrence deposits were known to exist since 1870 (Howley and Murray 1881, 235), but it was not until the 1920s, in conjunction with a growing demand for the mineral, that they attracted attention for their potential commercial value. In 1930, St. John's businessman John H. Taylor sold several claims he had staked in the area to Walter Seibert, a twenty-seven-year-old broker with the Corporation Trust Company of New York. After first trying to sell the claims, Seibert contacted St. Lawrence merchant Aubrey Farrell to arrange the mining and export of a 2,000-ton trial shipment. Under this arrangement, Seibert would supply the equipment and Farrell would receive a share of any profit. The workers would be paid fifteen cents an hour once the fluorspar was mined, shipped, sold, and paid for. In March 1933, a boat-load of dilapidated mining equipment, described by an

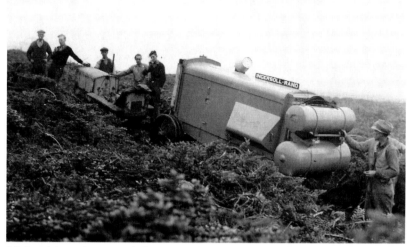

Moving mining equipment over the barrens, c. 1937.

industry observer as "second-hand junk, which would be discarded by any up-to-date mining concern,"[2] arrived in St. Lawrence. The people of the town unloaded the equipment and hauled it over the barrens to the "Black Duck" vein. The initial work of transporting and setting up the equipment was not part of the Seibert-Farrell arrangement; it was undertaken in the hope of paying work in the future. With Seibert's used equipment and a few basic hand tools, thirty men began mining the Black Duck vein and hauling the ore by horse and cart to a loading wharf in the community to be shipped to the Dominion Steel and Coal Corporation (Dosco) plant in Sydney, Nova Scotia (Martin 1983, 66–67; Farrell Edwards 1983, 70–71; Fischer and Howse 1939; Slaney 1975, 2–4). Farrell and men received payment more than a year after the initial deal was struck, and Seibert then formed the St. Lawrence Corporation of Newfoundland and hired a number of local men, former fishermen, to continue mining the Black Duck and other veins.[3]

"Treated Like a Bunch of Coolies"

The ore produced in the initial phase of mining was exceptionally pure, requiring only sorting and washing to bring it up to metallurgical grade.[4] Initially the veins were mined by the "open-cut" method: the vein was exposed from the surface and then followed vertically and horizontally as far as equipment and conditions would allow. The lack of proper equipment, however, made for arduous work, and conditions were treacherous as the trenches became deeper.[5] Miners had nothing in the way of safety clothing or basic facilities. In bad weather, they ate in small, unheated shacks used to house mining equipment or in the nearby woods. There were no bathroom

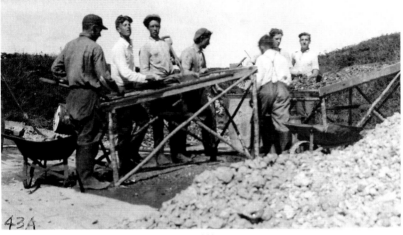

Young workers sorting ore at Black Duck mine, c. 1937.

facilities; workers simply went to the woods or stayed in the pit. Their drinking water came from streams or from the mine walls. Miners climbed wood ladders up and down the pits (Slaney 1975, 16–19) and by 1936, they were working in narrow trenches more than a hundred feet deep without proper hoisting or safety equipment of any kind.[6]

There was little to protect workers from such hazards. The establishment and expansion of copper mining on the island's northeast coast during the last half of the nineteenth century had prompted the suggestion, in 1877, that legislation be introduced to govern health and safety in mines, but nothing came of the proposal (Newfoundland 1877, 123). A similar suggestion ten years later met the same fate (Newfoundland 1887). In 1908, after the demise of those copper mines, legislation governing health and safety in mines was passed, mainly in response to the high accident rate at the iron ore mines that had been established at Bell Island, near St. John's, in 1895. The 1908 Act established standards in such areas as ventilation, explosives, hoisting, signaling devices, and tramways. However, inspections were conducted by the government engineer, who had no particular expertise in the area, and only in response to a fatal or serious accident (Newfoundland 1909). The shortcomings of this system were summed up by a Bell Island miner who remarked in 1912 that inspections were only conducted when another "mangled corpse" was brought out of the mine (*Daily News* February 19, 1912).

The government of the day showed little inclination to alter the status quo. Newfoundland was at that time run by a Commission of Government, appointed on the recommendation of a British Royal Commission whose "Amulree" report of 1933 described Newfoundland as crippled by widespread unemployment; inadequate medical, transportation and communication infrastructure; a stifling and exploitative merchant-credit system in the fishery; and a political environment marred by corruption (Lord Amulree 1933; Alexander 1976a; Neary 1988, 12–43). The Commission's most radical recommendation for responding to this situation was the suspension of Responsible Government (which had been in place since 1855) and the appointment of a Commission of Government to run the affairs of the colony until the situation had improved to the point where some form of elected government could be reinstated.

In January 1934 a Commission of Government — an unelected body of administrators and bureaucrats — was appointed to fulfill this role. The Commission of Government was divided into six departments — Finance, Justice, Home Affairs and Education, Public Utilities, Natural Resources, and Public Health and Welfare — and a Commissioner appointed to oversee each. Sir John Hope Simpson, a British civil servant with ample experience in responding to crises in such places as China and India, was appointed Commissioner of Natural Resources, which included mines. The Health and Welfare portfolio, which included labour, went to John. C. Puddester, who had served as minister of that department in the last administration under Responsible Government (Neary 1988, 44–52; Noel 1971, 202–43).

When the District Magistrate drew his attention to conditions at the mines in March 1936, the Commissioner of Natural Resources simply replied that the mine he had visited in 1935 had seemed very dangerous at the time but he had since been assured that it was "perfectly safe." The only substantial aspect of the response was a concern that the St. Lawrence Corporation might lack the capital to fully develop the resource and a suggestion that the government secure a loan of $150,000 to be used in upgrading and expanding operations.[7] Nothing came of the suggestion, but it clearly illustrates the government's priorities. Furthermore, the exchange underscores the fact that the structure of the Commission of Government left it unclear exactly who was responsible for occupational health and safety — certainly not Natural Resources.

Shortly after the Magistrate drew attention to the St. Lawrence situation, the Geological Division of the Department of Natural Resources pointed out that since approximately 2,500 men were now employed in mining around the island, a full-time mines inspector might be required.[8] The 2,500 included a hundred at St. Lawrence, 1,800 at the Bell Island iron mines, and the remainder at a lead, zinc and copper mine established by an American firm at Buchans, in the island's interior, in 1927. Again the Commissioner saw little cause for concern, noting that there had been "only" five fatal accidents in Newfoundland mines during the preceding year (1935).[9] Before long Hope Simpson was replaced as Commissioner of Natural Resources by Robert Ewbank, who agreed that there was no need to employ a full-time inspector and that "negotiations to this end might be dropped."[10]

While he rejected calls for a full-time inspector, Ewbank did bring in an inspector from Ontario, a step he described as a temporary solution until the Department of Public Utilities assumed responsibility for health and safety in the mines.[11] When A.E. Cave of the Ontario Department of Mines conducted the first ever general inspection of Newfoundland mines, in August 1939, five mines were operating at St. Lawrence, the largest of them Black Duck and Iron Springs. Cave described methods at all sites as "primitive." Though there were a few air compressors and jackhammers in use, much of the work was done by hand. Cave's main concerns were the potential for cave-ins and flooding in the open cuts, and the lack of toilet facilities and clean drinking water. He also had suggestions regarding the use of explosives, hauling and hoisting devices, safety belts, and other matters. On a more general level, he recommended that the government hire a qualified inspector to carry out regular, detailed inspections and that it require mining companies to submit mine plans and the details of all fatalities and injuries, a requirement that was routine in jurisdictions across Canada.[12] The government took no action in response to these suggestions.

The government's refusal to address the inadequate health and safety regime was compounded by its policies regarding public relief. From its inception in 1934, the government focused on reducing both the number of people on public relief and the amounts distributed to recipients, an effort driven by the inadequacy of the system and growing financial demand. Historically, the relief system in Newfoundland had been administered by the central government on an ad hoc basis and was intended primarily to meet the needs of the infirm, the aged, widows, and others who could not look after themselves and had no family or other support. With about 30 percent of the population on public relief in some areas, even during the fishing season,[13] the system was under intense financial and administrative pressure (Overton 1994, 79–122).

The Commission of Government itself was also under pressure from the Dominions Office, as the British government required the Commission to submit frequent, detailed reports on public relief, justify all expenditures, and explain any increase in relief numbers.[14] This demand arose partly from political realities within Great Britain where, with the situation at home also desperate, the government was forced to explain expenditures in a distant former colony. In 1934, for instance, an official with the Dominions Office noted that information on the employment situation in Newfoundland would help answer some potentially "awkward" questions in Parliament.[15]

In response to these combined pressures, the Commission essentially adopted the approach that had evolved in Great Britain. There, by the early 1930s, the unemployed had been divided into two general groups: the temporarily unemployed, who were insured for a given period, and the long-term unemployed, who were subject to a means test to qualify for state assistance. The latter group included many able-bodied unemployed who were required to meet certain conditions to qualify for assistance, including proof that they had sought employment and not turned down any employment offered to them (Garside 1990, 32–65). This approach institutionalized the distinction between the "deserving" and the "undeserving" poor, and strengthened a long-standing feature of the British system, the principle of "less eligibility," under which those receiving public relief were to be kept at a living standard below that of the lowest paid worker. Public relief was thus designed to be so unattractive as to compel persons to seek and retain almost any kind of employment. During the Depression, the government of Great Britain became more proactive in this regard, adopting measures to force all "voluntary unemployed back into the labour market" (Whiteside 1991, 83). In the Canadian public relief system during the 1930s, as well, a chief aim was to "preserve the motivation of those who worked, particularly those in the worst jobs society had to offer" (Struthers 1983, 6–7).

To maintain strict control over the public relief system in Newfoundland, the Commission of Government's Department of Public Health and Welfare set strict guidelines for granting and administering relief. Officials were ordered to investigate every claim, to issue relief only when and to whom it was absolutely necessary, and to distribute the absolute minimum.[16] Officials were also warned to be wary of "slackers" who refused or abandoned work on "the usual flimsy pretexts of unpleasant or unremunerative activities."[17]

The St. Lawrence Corporation used this system to drive down the price of labour and quash potential unrest. For example, in 1936 the company offered a group of their regular employees sixty cents per ton to haul ore from a mine site to the dock for shipment. When the men objected to the wage, the company offered the work to unemployed men on relief, who could not refuse the work at any wage offered, since they would then be cut from the relief roll.[18] The degree of power wielded by the company under the circumstances is illustrated in another incident recalled by Richard Clarke, who started work as an ore-sorter in 1936, when he was sixteen years old:

> One time when we were picking the ore… Kelleher [the American manager brought in by Seibert] was the manager then of the St. Lawrence Corporation. This morning the boys… we all left the job and came out and wanted more pay, so we went down and went in talking to old Kelleher and he was pretty upset and he said, "Well boys, I'll tell you what I'll do for you… if you don't go back to work now any one of you that got your father working in the mine I'll lay off you and I'll lay off your father too. And we had to go back and go to work…. No choice.[19]

Conditions at St. Lawrence grew markedly worse from late 1936, when shafts were sunk and operations moved underground at various sites.[20] Once underground mining began, two basic methods were used to extract ore, "benching" and "open-stoping." With each method, horizontal tunnels or "drifts" were established at various depths along the shaft, parallel to the vein. With the benching method, workers drilled and blasted the ore to create a series of downward terraces at intervals along a drift. With stoping, which would become the most common method used at St. Lawrence, workers also drilled and blasted ore at intervals along the drift, but instead of "benching down," they proceeded inward and upward. Ore was blasted from the vein but, rather than being removed right away, this broken ore, or "muck," was left for miners to work from as they proceeded inward and upward. If stoping was carried out to a sufficient height, the stope would eventually break through to the level above, creating a honeycomb pattern of horizontal and vertical openings throughout the mine. The ore was then shovelled into tram cars that were rolled along tracks through the drift and dumped down "ore passes" into a collection point known as a "loading pocket," from which it was hoisted in the ore bucket, or "skip," to the surface.

While it provided some shelter from the elements, the move underground made hazards more frequent and more serious. One of the first to work underground at the Black Duck mine recalled:

> Before this, in the open cut, dust and smoke were not so much of a problem…. In the [underground], drilling was done with a dry hammer. This machine was second-hand and had already drilled thousands of feet on some other job. The hammer was hung on the shoulder which brought the drill hole directly opposite the driller's

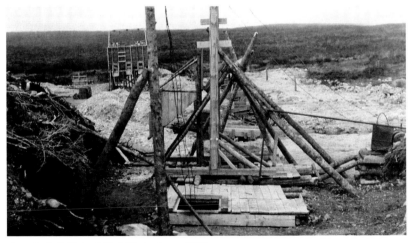

An early shaft, likely at Black Duck mine, c. 1937.

mouth…. He also, at times, used curtain screen or cheesecloth over his mouth, but this clogged with dust in seconds and had to be discarded. Every few minutes, he would have to shut off the machine to clear his eyes and nostrils of dust…. The further the drifts advanced, the dust and smoke became worse. (Slaney 1975, 14–15)

These "dry drills" were among the pieces of used equipment Seibert had shipped to St. Lawrence in 1933 and were so called to distinguish them from the more modern "axial" type, also available at the time, that supplied a flow of water to the drill bit to suppress dust. Dry drills, known as "widow-makers" among early twentieth-century silver miners in Northern Ontario, had long been recognized as hazardous to health because of the dust they generated. As early as 1913, the Ontario government recognized the danger "arising from the breathing of the dust… from the hammer drills where no water is used to allay the dust," and the Ontario Mines Act was amended in 1914 to address this hazard. After that water-fed drills gradually replaced dry drills in Ontario mines (Baldwin 1977, 92–93). Wet drills were also standard equipment in the fluorspar mines of Kentucky and Illinois by the 1920s (Fellman 1926, 206; Rosner 1992, 135–54). The fact that dry drills had been discarded and outlawed in many North American jurisdictions by the 1930s suggests why Seibert was able to purchase some well-used ones to ship to St. Lawrence.

By 1937, workers were sufficiently incensed by the situation to stage a brief walkout to protest working conditions and the method of wage payment. These grievances were put to the Government Geologist, Claude Howse, who was in St. Lawrence to offer advice to a second company that planned to start mining there. This company was formed by a partnership between a St. John's manufacturer who held a number of mineral claims in the area and E.J. Lavino and Company, a Philadelphia-based firm involved in the production and distribution of mineral and chemical products. Exploration work carried out by this newly formed company, the American-Newfoundland Fluorspar Corporation (ANF), had revealed two large veins of ore, the "Director" and the "Tarefare" veins (Martin 1983, 70; Fischer and Howse 1939).

The town's merchants complained to Howse that since there were often insufficient funds in the company's bank account to cover paycheques, workers were forced to take up credit at the stores and were constantly in debt. Kelleher suggested that workers had little grounds for complaint as their jobs were better than the only alternative, public relief. The Parish Priest had reportedly "done his best in keeping the men contented and optimistic," and "smoothed over whatever trouble and contention there has appeared in the past." Howse inspected the mines and found that Black Duck shaft was flooded up to thirty-five feet at the base, a highly dangerous condition.[21]

According to Howse, workers had been prepared to put up with substandard conditions in the beginning in the hope that things would improve, but were "gradually leaning to the opinion that Seibert is using them as pawns and cares absolutely nothing about the welfare of the men."[22] One merchant put the situation in stark terms when he noted in a letter to his St. John's wholesaler that "the people are treated like a bunch of coolies and have to accept it owing to the depression and nothing else to earn."[23] The supplier forwarded the letter to Ewbank, who brought it to Seibert's attention. However, Ewbank was less than firm in his demands: he told Seibert that Government was "concerned" with the state of affairs and asked him what he intended to do about it.[24]

That the government ignored obvious problems and grievances is perhaps not surprising given its overriding concern with reducing public relief expenditure and maintaining all avenues of employment. Shortly after the 1937 walkout, a Public Relief report noted that

> ...the two mining companies operating at St. Lawrence are absorbing practically all the able-bodied labor available. Rates and conditions do not appear to be very satisfactory, but the men are at least self-supporting. If the work does cease or if it is curtailed to any material extent, much destitution will almost certainly prevail with consequent large demands on us for public relief.[25]

Meanwhile, as underground mining advanced, conditions grew more hazardous. Flooding and other problems forced the Iron Springs operation underground in 1938, and conditions there were reported to be even worse than those at Black Duck. The Iron Springs vein was exceptionally rich but also very narrow, intensifying the problems of dust, smoke, and inadequate ventilation. Richard Clarke, who worked underground at Iron Springs in the late 1930s, recalled that there was "no ventilation at all whatsoever" and that the dust was "in your mouth and falling out of your hair and you could feel it grinding under your teeth."[26]

Growing Fears and Getting Organized

The effects of these working conditions were becoming apparent by the late 1930s. In the summer of 1939, nearly all of the St. Lawrence Corporation's hundred workers were suffering from stomach ailments, which the Department of Public Health and Welfare later attributed to the "a high state of pollution" found in water samples taken underground.[27]

It was in this context that workers began taking a more organized approach to their efforts and that the dependence and powerlessness characteristic of labour relations in the 1930s began to change. Coinciding with the outbreak of illness, workers organized the St. Lawrence Miners and Labourers Protective Union (SLMLPU). The president of the SLMLPU was a local merchant named Patrick Aylward.[28] Aylward later claimed that he had been approached by several miners during the summer of 1939 to help form a union. It is unclear why he was chosen for this task, as Aylward seems to have had no experience with either mining or unionism. It is possible that the absence of any tradition of unionism in the area, combined with the lack of local government, left workers with few options when it came to leadership figures. Aylward may also have been one of the few local men, apart from the priest and a few school teachers, who were literate.

The decision to unionize represented a significant break with tradition for a workforce composed largely of former fishermen with no direct experience in organized labour. Viewed in a wider context, however, the establishment of the SLMLPU can be seen as part of a trend taking place across Newfoundland at the time. While the harsh economic circumstances of the 1930s may have stifled workers' ability to engage in organizing and unrest, by mid-decade they may have occasionally had the opposite effect. For example, Newfoundland loggers, who for years had endured some of the worst living and working conditions on the island, organized in 1934 under the Newfoundland Loggers' Association and were soon engaged in a series of strikes and protests (Sutherland 1992, 81–116). In the same year, Buchans miners formed the Buchans Workers Protective Union (BWPU) with an initial membership of four hundred (Gillespie 1986, 63–64). The formation of the Newfoundland Trades and Labour Council (NTLC) in 1936 resulted from and further fuelled this trend. Largely as a result of the NTLC's efforts, total union membership in Newfoundland tripled from 1936 to 1939 and on the eve of the Second World War Newfoundland had one of the highest rates of unionization in all of North America (Kealey 1986, 113, 16).

The Commission of Government, like previous administrations, had no department or staff specifically dedicated to labour issues. Given the economic situation when it took office, the government likely believed it had little cause to fear labour unrest, and labour matters had simply been subsumed under the Department of Public Utilities. The lack of dedicated resources and a coherent policy in this area would have a strong influence on the interaction of the state, employers, and workers across Newfoundland, including at St. Lawrence.

By the end of 1939, the SLMLPU had issued several demands to the St. Lawrence Corporation for improvements in working conditions, particularly with respect to drinking water and sanitation.[29] To this the management responded with paternalism or obstinacy. At Christmas, for instance, the company announced a 10 percent wage increase, described as "a Xmas box," for all employees. One observer applauded this move on the grounds that it was "voluntary" and thus contributed to "the happy relations so much to be desired between capital and labour" (*Evening Telegram* January 5, 1940). Others were less impressed: an anonymous letter-writer (possibly Aylward) suggested that the raise was a response to the formation of the union and an attempt to put a good public face on a bad situation (*Evening Telegram* February 1, 1940).

The pay raise also did nothing to address ongoing health concerns. In the first instance of a specific industrial disease being mentioned as a possibility among St. Lawrence miners, in January 1940 the Department of Public Health and Welfare expressed fear that possible cases of lung diseases, such as silicosis, were beginning to surface in the copper mines at Buchans and that similar problems might exist at St. Lawrence.[30] Whether aware of it or not, the Department of Public Health and Welfare had good grounds for this suspicion. The St. Lawrence mines were an ideal environment for silicosis to take hold, since it is caused by the inhalation of fine dust created by drilling hard rock, such as the granite that surrounds the St. Lawrence fluorspar veins (Webster 1972, 20–38; Derickson 1988a, 180–81; 1988b; Collis and Greenwood 1977, 144; Parkinson 1955; Gibbs and Pintus 1978, 84, 95–99; James 1993).

In noting the possibility of illnesses linked to working conditions, the Department of Public Health and Welfare pointed out that in the absence of any effective legislation the government could do little but hope that the companies involved would look after such matters out of concern for their workers. However, the Department was apparently not convinced that mine operators would voluntarily show such concern, and urged the Department of Justice to amend the Public Health and Welfare Act to cover conditions at mines and other industrial sites, since as it stood the legislation applied only to logging camps.[31]

Concerns about possible silicosis and the fear that "the unsanitary surroundings and unhealthy water supplies" might cause an outbreak of disease[32] were compounded by the fact that there was no hospital or doctor in St. Lawrence. The 1933 Amulree Commission had noted the lack of medical services in the country, pointing out that there were just four hospitals outside St. John's and just sixty-two physicians to serve some 1,300 settlements scattered around the coast (Lord Amulree 1933, 592–93). In an attempt to address this problem, the Commission of Government introduced a program in 1934 to construct and staff hospitals around the island. Of the thirteen new facilities established under this initiative by the end of the Second World War, the nearest to St. Lawrence was one that opened in the late 1930s at Burin, the commercial and administrative centre of the region, about thirty kilometres away (MacKay 1946, 178–79). However, there was no road linking St. Lawrence directly to Burin until the 1950s, and travel between the two towns was undertaken on foot, by boat, or by horse and sled. A road that ran out of St. Lawrence in the opposite direction looped back around to Burin, but this route was about 150 kilometres of rough road, impassable in winter. According to the Department of Public Health and Welfare, the St. Lawrence Corporation had been approached for assistance in establishing medical facilities at St. Lawrence, but had been "absolutely non-cooperative."[33]

Some workers at St. Lawrence also suspected that conditions in the mines were damaging their health, but were uncertain exactly how. Richard Clarke recalled, "After you'd get there for a couple of months, you'd start losing your appetite and the strength would go, you'd start losing the strength in your legs, and you'd find it hard to breathe."[34] Clarke was one of those who escaped the impending disaster. He worked in the mines during the winter for a few years but continued to fish as his chief livelihood, and eventually got out of mining altogether. Many others would not be as fortunate.

Notes

1. Report of the Receiving Officer for Lamaline,12 March 1936, GN 38, S6-1-1, File 7, PANL; and Magistrate's Report to the Department of Natural Resources, 31 July 1936, GN38, S4-3-3, File 7, PANL.
2. Letter from C. Wilbur Miller of Dupont Chemicals to Lammot Dupont, 11 February 1937, Files of the Hagley Museum and Library, Wilmington, Delaware.
3, W.S. Smith, Fluorspar at St. Lawrence, 1957, Archival Collection of Newfoundland and Labrador Department of Mines and Energy (hereafter DME).
4. C.K. Howse, The Fluorspar Industry at St. Lawrence, 1936, File 1L/14 (3), DME.
5. C.K. Howse, The Fluorspar Industry at St. Lawrence, 1936, File 1L/14 (3), DME.
6. Magistrate's Report to the Department of Natural Resources, 25 March 1936, GN38, S2-1-11, File 1, PANL.
7. Memorandum submitted by Commissioner for Natural Resources for Consideration of Commission of Government, 16 April 1936, GN 38, S2-1-11, File 1, PANL.
8. Proposal that the operator of the diamond drill should be competent to inspect mines and also the matter of financial provision therefor, 26 May 1936, GN 38, S1-1-12, File 8 (NR 63-36), PANL.
9. Proposal that the operator of the diamond drill should be competent to inspect mines and also the matter of financial provision therefor, 26 May 1936, GN 38, S1-1-12, File 8 (NR 63-36), PANL.
10. Memorandum re Inspection of Mines in Newfoundland, 4 July 1936, GN38, S-1-12, File 18 (NR 63b-36), PANL.
11. Memorandum re Inspection of Mines in Newfoundland, 4 July 1936, GN38, S-1-12, File 18 (NR 63b-36), PANL.

12. A.E. Cave, Report on Mines Inspection of Newfoundland, Submitted to Newfoundland Commission of Government, Department of Natural Resources, 6 November 1936, DME.

13. Records of the Dominions Office (hereafter DO), 35/499/Pt. 2/1934.

14. Thomas Lodge, Commissioner for Public Utilities, to P.A. Clutterbuck, Dominions Office, 19 October 1934, DO 35/499/N1028/4.

15. P.A. Clutterbuck, Dominions Office, to Thomas Lodge, Commissioner for Public Utilities, 19 October, 1934, DO35/499, CNS.

16. Memorandum on dole operations, 15 December 1934, GN38, S6-1-1, File 2 (PHW 6-35/36), PANL, and Memorandum regarding the supply of clothing relief to the outports during the coming winter, 30 October 1935, GN38, S6-1-1, File 2 (PHW 48-34), PANL.

17. Report on the relief situation on the Burin Peninsula and the south coast, August 1937, GN38, S6-1-2, File 4, PANL.

18. Magistrate's Report to the Department of Natural Resources, 25 March 1936, GN38, S2-1-11, File 1, PANL.

19. Interview with Richard Clarke, 26 October 1997.

20. C.K. Howse, The Fluorspar Industry at St. Lawrence, 1936, File 1L/14 (3), DME.

21. Report on Investigation of Conditions at St. Lawrence, 8 June 1937, GN38, S-1-11, File 1 (NR 44-37), PANL.

22. Report on Investigation of Conditions at St. Lawrence, 8 June 1937, GN38, S-1-11, File 1 (NR 44-37), PANL.

23. L.J. Saint, St. Lawrence to Stephenson, Royal Stores, St. John's, 9 June 1937, GN 38, S1-11, File 1 (NR 44-37), PANL.

24. Department of Natural Resources to Mr. W.E. Seibert, St. Lawrence Corporation, Nutley, N,J, GN38, S-1-11, File 1, (NR44-37), PANL.

25. Report on the relief situation on the Burin Peninsula and the south coast, August 1937, GN38, S6-1-2, File 4, PANL.

26. Interview with Richard Clarke, 26 October 1997.

27. Memorandum respecting the report by Dr. J. St. P. Knight, 4 December 1939, PANL, GN38, S-6-1-2, File 12.

28. Report made by Magistrate Short on the subject of a dispute between the St. Lawrence Corporation of Newfoundland Ltd., and the St. Lawrence Miners and Labourers Protective Union, 23 May 1940, PANL, GN38, S5-4-1, File 5.

29. Ranger V.P. Duff's Report on Conditions at the Fluorspar Mine, St. Lawrence, 5 December 1939, PANL, GN38, S6-1-2, File 40.

30. Department of Public Health and Welfare to Department of Natural Resources, 15 January 1940, PANL, GN38, S6-1-2, File 40.

31. Department of Public Health and Welfare to Department of Justice, 15 December 1939, PANL, GN38, S6-2-1, File 12.

32. Department of Public Health and Welfare to Department of Natural Resources, 15 January 1940, PANL, GN38, S6-1-2, File 40.

33. Department of Public Health and Welfare to Department of Natural Resources, 15 January 1940 PANL, GN38, S6-1-2, File 40.

34. Interview with Richard Clarke, 26 October 1997.

Chapter Two

PROTEST AND RETREAT
The War Years

Industry Expansion and Increasing Strength

While unionization increased the potential for workers to take collective action on their complaints, what put them in position to use that potential was
increased demand for fluorspar, industry expansion, and a general economic
upswing during the early years of the Second World War. At the end of the
1930s, the ore from the St. Lawrence Corporation mines was still used in
steel manufacturing and the main buyer was still Dosco. However, rising
demand for aluminum in the United States, Great Britain, and Canada
brought an increased need for smelting agents such as fluorspar, prompting
Canada's chief producer, the Aluminum Company of Canada (Alcan), to
expand its smelting facilities and seek new sources of raw material (Campbell
1985, 333–34; Brubaker 1967, 101–23). Alcan looked to St. Lawrence as a
source for its smelter at Arvida, Quebec, and in December 1939 acquired
the properties held by the ANF and formed a subsidiary, Newfoundland
Fluorspar Limited, or "Newfluor."[1] By early 1940, Newfluor had hired fifty
men to work the Director vein, with the intention of going into production
by the summer of that year.[2]

Expansion at the St. Lawrence Corporation, driven by increased demand for fluorspar at Dosco, had increased the workforce to about 150
when workers there walked off the job in April 1940 in another attempt to
force action on long-standing grievances.[3] Testimony given at a magistrate's
inquiry into the walkout reveals how changes in the economic environment
had both improved workers' ability to take action and intensified hazards
in the workplace. Union president Aylward stated that the workers had escaped the "dread of poverty" that had prevented them from complaining
more forcefully in the past. Some concerns Aylward listed had been raised
previously, including no sanitation facilities or clean drinking water and
dangerous hoisting equipment. However, he also noted that the expansion of
underground mining had intensified the problem of inadequate ventilation,
and he reported several cases of "suffocation."

Workers substantiated Aylward's claims. One stated that his only source
of drinking water was from a hose that supplied water to cool the underground equipment. Another claimed that in the Iron Springs shaft the only
source of ventilation was the hoses that provided compressed air to the ma-

chinery, which workers periodically removed to breathe from. The same man also recalled an incident in which a worker had to be revived with air from a hose when he passed out underground. Asked whose responsibility it was to monitor ventilation and other health and safety matters at the mines, he replied that he did not know. Another miner stated: "We have no ventilation in our mine," and reported that two men had recently fainted underground for lack of air.

Others testified that the manager, Donald Poynter (an American who had been brought in by Seibert to replace Kelleher), had threatened to fire them if they complained about working conditions. One worker recalled complaining to his foreman that his task was too much for one man, only to be told that if he could not do the work he could easily be replaced. Another testified that he was fired because he had complained to the union about working conditions, and he reported being later told by the manager, "Well, you had a bad back and you're getting old…. [You are] no good for the mine any more."[4]

Not surprisingly, Poynter presented a very different picture. He denied that the company had threatened or taken disciplinary action against men who had complained of working conditions.[5] Poynter did not dispute the claims regarding sanitary conditions but attempted to deflect criticism away from the company by denigrating miners' homes:

> Sanitary arrangements, drinking water arrangements, and conditions under which men work are in my opinion equal to, if not better than they have in their own homes. When the time comes when St. Lawrence will take an interest in its own sanitation and drinking water and show evidence of this interest in their own homes, this Company will gladly give them the equal in their working conditions.[6]

Regarding the issue of ventilation in the mines, Poynter stated that it was "more than adequate" and added a vague assurance that "The entire ventilation scheme of this mine is following a definite plan that was conceived by a trained engineer."[7]

Poynter also denied that the St. Lawrence Corporation opposed the formation of the union, but correspondence produced at the inquiry revealed that the company refused to recognize the union as a bargaining agent for its employees. For instance, in response to a request from the union in October 1939 that official communications be established between the two parties, Poynter had stated that he would discuss company-employee relations only with individual workers.[8] Several months later, Aylward made the same request to Seibert and received no reply.[9]

Union recognition was a vexing issue, for while Newfoundland's Trade

Union Act, passed in 1910, protected the right of workers to unionize, it did not compel employers to recognize the union. Canadian unions faced a similar problem, and as one historian has noted, the legislation failed to account for the fact that recognition is unlike other collective bargaining issues, since "the very existence of one of the parties was not an issue for which there was a middle ground" (MacDowell 1978, 179).

In the event, the April 1940 walkout and the ensuing inquiry did little to advance the workers' cause. The magistrate's report to government failed to mention any of the specific issues raised by Aylward and the workers. Instead, the report focused on the actions of the union, concluding that it had been confrontational in its approach and created an antagonistic environment.[10]

Nor was there much indication that the situation would be improved through government action on health and safety. In June 1940, two months after the magistrate's inquiry, A.E. Cave of the Ontario Department of Mines toured the mines of Newfoundland for a second time. At this time the shafts at both Iron Springs and Black Duck were down to about 200 feet, while Newfluor's Director shaft was down to 150 feet. Most of Cave's recommendations focused on safety hazards, including hoisting practices, explosives, rockfalls, and escape routes, but he also pointed to the need for clean drinking water and toilet facilities. Cave also reiterated his 1936 observations about the inadequacy of the Newfoundland regulations and repeated his recommendation that the government establish a regular inspection service.[11] Once again, the government took no action on the proposals.

Escalating Conflict and Demands for State Intervention

Having made no progress on its demands under Aylward's leadership of the SLMLPU, the membership ousted Aylward in January 1941 and dissolved the union. Aylward was replaced by union treasurer Aloysius Turpin. Unlike Aylward, Turpin was drawn from the membership, having worked as a miner and a carpenter for the St. Lawrence Corporation. He would go on to become a central and sometimes controversial figure in the union and its actions. The membership also reconstituted the union as the St. Lawrence Workers Protective Union (SLWPU). As an indication of the climate of fear that marked the labour relations environment at the time, Turpin recalled that workers had waited until Poynter went to New York before calling the meeting at which these changes were made.[12]

The SLWPU wasted little time in pressing its demands. On March 17, 1941, just two days after the union was formed, workers at both the St. Lawrence Corporation and Newfluor walked off the job in a dispute ostensibly about whether or not St. Patrick's Day would be observed as a holiday.[13] While this was of some significance to the mostly Catholic workforce, it appears to have served mainly as an issue over which the new union and its leader could assert themselves. It is unclear how the matter of a St. Patrick's Day holiday was settled, but the men returned to work after just two days.

About a month later, however, St. Lawrence Corporation workers walked off the job again over wages and working conditions.[14] The union was also protesting the St. Lawrence Corporation's continued refusal to recognize it as the members' bargaining agent, and alleging that the company was still engaged in anti-union tactics.[15] Newfluor had already agreed to recognize the SLWPU as the sole bargaining agent for its employees.[16] The St. Lawrence Corporation, however, would agree only to recognizing the union as "the bargaining agent of members who are our employees," which did not satisfy the union as it excluded several workers who had not yet joined the union.[17] After a week the men again agreed to return to work and the union then drafted a collective agreement that included a demand for employment of union members only as well as for compensation for disabled workers.

The demand for compensation benefits underscores the status of Newfoundland's workers' compensation system at the time, which had remained unchanged since the Workmen's Compensation Act of 1908. The 1908 Act required employers to pay compensation directly to injured workers (or in the case of death, their dependents) once claimants had either come to a private arrangement with the employer or had the claim settled in court (Newfoundland 1909b). The Newfoundland system thus retained some elements of the Common Law system that had prevailed there as well as in Britain and Canada until the early twentieth century, most notably in the involvement of the courts and in the paying of benefits by employers directly to claimants. This differed from the British Act introduced in 1906, which did not involve the courts and which required employers to pay premiums into a collective fund, which was then used to pay claims. By 1930 all Canadian provinces but Prince Edward Island had introduced legislation based on the British model (Prince Edward Island did so in 1949) (Logan 1948, 501; Piva 1975, 39–56). Because under this arrangement employers' premiums were based on their record of compensable injuries and illnesses, the system was also intended to have a protective component, providing a financial incentive to protect workers' health and safety. In Great Britain and in Canada many employers supported the legislation because they believed such a system would ultimately result in lower costs to them and because it removed the right of claimants to sue them (Reasons et al. 1981, 163–64). Newfoundland would not make the transition to a modern system until after confederation with Canada in 1949. According to a committee that later studied the matter, very few claims were ever made under the pre-Confederation system and most were "settled by compromise [private arrangement], usually to the detriment of the worker" (Fogwill 1950, 2–3).

Another important aspect of the draft collective agreement the union presented to the St. Lawrence Corporation in 1941 was a demand that "the present unhealthy form of equipment[,] namely the Dry Jack Hammer[,]" be abolished and replaced by "proper wet drills." The union also requested the establishment of a Safety Committee with an equal number of union and company representatives, with the power to investigate working conditions and make recommendations to management, as well as a provision to have an outside authority decide on any health and safety matter on which this committee could not reach agreement.[18] This proposed agreement was forwarded to the Public Utilities Commissioner, along with a request for the appointment of a "Board of Enquiry." The union agreed to continue production pending the appointment of such an inquiry.[19]

The Commission of Government's response to this request and to subsequent developments at St. Lawrence must be viewed in the context of its general response to labour unrest. The issue of the government's lack of a legislative framework or a coherent policy in the area of labour became more pressing when Newfoundland was drawn into the Second World War alongside Great Britain in the fall of 1939, since the need to maintain production in vital industries coupled with an increased demand for labour threatened to generate further labour unrest. While the government had ample power to intervene in labour disputes under wartime measures passed in 1939, it initially chose instead to pursue a combination of damage control and ad hoc measures.

At one point, after having to appoint a committee to settle a strike by St. John's longshoremen in January 1940, the Commission of Government did consider adopting legislation modelled on the Canadian Industrial Disputes Investigation Act (IDIA) of 1907, which included provisions for compulsory investigation of labour disputes by a government-appointed third party and prohibition of work stoppages pending such investigation (Neary 1988, 169). However, the government soon abandoned this route and reverted to its piecemeal approach.

Increased pressure came to bear when a deal was struck in the fall of 1940 to allow for the establishment of American and Canadian military bases at several sites around the island. In January 1941, the first legions of American servicemen began to arrive, and soon an estimated 20,000 Newfoundland civilians were employed in the construction of military bases. Combined with the wartime revival of many other industries (such as shipping, mining, and forestry), the so-called "base-building boom" created an unprecedented demand for labour and a serious concern for the government. Government now had to deal with the combined threat of a revitalized labour movement and the spectre of two foreign governments exporting their standards of work practices and remuneration to Newfoundland. Public Utilities Commissioner Wilfrid Woods described the situation as a "golden opportunity" for the growth and spread of trade unions and for increased labour militancy.[20] Woods was soon proven right, as beginning in early 1941 workers both on and off the bases used a variety of channels to demand improvements in working conditions and wages.

The government's response to the SLWPU's request for a government inquiry in May of 1941 was in keeping with its desultory approach to that point: Woods proposed a meeting among representatives of the union, the St. Lawrence Corporation, and the government the next time Seibert visited from New York.[21] Turpin refused the invitation, telling Woods that while he had managed to keep the men working to this point, they had vowed nothing short of an official government inquiry would satisfy them. The main issues the union wanted addressed by such an inquiry were health and safety and union recognition.[22]

This second request for government intervention came shortly after the Commission of Government adopted measures that specifically included the power to intervene in labour disputes. The Defence (Avoidance of Strikes and Lockouts) Regulations gave the government several options in the event of a real or threatened strike or lockout, including the establishment of a tribunal, the outright prohibition of a strike or lockout, the imposition of terms and conditions of work upon employers, and the power to change any rule or accepted practice with respect to conditions of employment (Newfoundland 1941b).

Woods, however, continued to delay formal intervention and wanted, "in the interests of all concerned," to meet with Seibert before taking any further action.[23] Turpin again warned Woods that the men would not work much longer under current conditions and insisted that they were asking only to be "treated as human beings."[24] Woods ignored the warning and held a meeting with Seibert, at which Seibert agreed to raise St. Lawrence Corporation wages to the level being paid at Newfluor. However, Seibert refused the union's demand to force the few non-union men still on the payroll to join the union or be dismissed from their jobs.[25] On the issue of health and safety, Seibert promised to "do our best to comply with the spirit and letter of all laws and regulations" and to do "everything within reason to better the health and working conditions of our employees."[26]

What the St. Lawrence Corporation considered "within reason" had given cause for doubt in the past. Even so, Woods seemed satisfied with Seibert's promise to raise wages and agreed with his position regarding the non-union men. He also rejected the request for an inquiry because Seibert had several objections to it, "into the merits of which I do not propose to enter now."[27] Refusing to conduct an inquiry because Seibert objected to it constituted a flagrant neglect of duty on Woods' part. Furthermore, Woods apparently believed that the important matters had been settled by Seibert's response to the issues of wages and the employment of non-union workers, a position that signalled his willingness to push health and safety concerns off the agenda and simply let the company's appeal to the existence of legislation substitute for concrete action in that area.

Although the union was not satisfied with Woods' most recent response to its demands, the men stayed on the job throughout the summer. In late August, however, their antagonism and resolve were hardened by the government's response to a labour dispute at Buchans, where earlier that month about seven hundred members of the Buchans Workers Protective Union had walked off the job over issues of wages and working conditions. While Woods initially avoided government intervention, in mid-August he gave in and appointed a tribunal under the Strikes and Lockouts Regulations. The Tribunal awarded the workers a cost-of-living wage increase but offered little meaningful response to the health and safety concerns raised by the union. Regarding complaints about dust and chemicals in the processing mill, for example, the Tribunal simply recommended that "a few respirators" be made available and that efforts be made to alleviate such hazards. "Apart from that," the Tribunal concluded, "we can only leave the matter to such mine inspections as may be possible from time to time" (Newfoundland 1941, 12–13).

Shortly after the Buchans settlement the SLWPU issued an ultimatum to Woods: guarantee appointment of an inquiry by September 15 or the men would go on strike.[28] Woods' response to this ultimatum was telling. First, he described difficulties at St. Lawrence as having arisen from two concerns: wage rates at the St. Lawrence Corporation and the employment of non-union labour. He was satisfied that both of these had been resolved.[29] Second, Woods worried that, "If this sort of thing is encouraged, there will have to be a Board appointed for every wage dispute and the Government will be burdened with the cost of a very considerable staff to form some sort of Labour Department," a concept that revealed yet another reason for the government's reluctance to become involved in labour relations matters in any systematic way.[30]

A month after the expiry of the deadline presented in the ultimatum, St. Lawrence Corporation workers walked off the job, protesting "unsatisfactory wage rates plus unhealthy and unsafe working conditions." The union also repeated its demands for recognition as the sole bargaining unit for employees of St. Lawrence Corporation.[31] At this point a standoff ensued. St. Lawrence Corporation manager Donald Poynter blamed the crisis on the union executive, motivated he claimed by "personal antagonism" rather than concern for the workers. He called upon the government to "step in and restrain these men," so that employees could return to work "unhampered by membership in this local union." Poynter also expressed confusion about the union's actions, pointing out that the St. Lawrence Corporation was now paying the same wage as Newfluor and "the question of safety is one that is covered by law."[32] The union, meanwhile, claimed that past dealings with the company had convinced workers that the only solution to the crisis was third-party intervention, and it vowed that the men would not return to work until an inquiry was established.[33]

The government continued to avoid intervening in the St. Lawrence situation while simultaneously bolstering its legislative power to do so. In the wake of a strike by St. John's longshoremen that threatened to withhold supplies to the American naval base in nearby Argentia, the government passed the Defence (Control and Conditions of Employment and Disputes Settlement) Regulations. These regulations gave the Commissioner for Public Utilities the power to appoint a Trade Dispute Board to settle disputes that affected "the defence of Newfoundland or the efficient prosecution of the war or maintaining supplies and services essential to the life of the community."[34]

Similar to the provisions of the Canadian IDIA, the regulations required that once a Trade Dispute Board had been appointed, any strike or lockout had to be suspended and work resumed pending the Board's rulings. A Board's decisions were to have the status of a contract, staying in effect "until varied by a subsequent agreement, decision or award."[35] While the new regulations had the potential to undermine the standard collective bargaining process, they could also benefit workers in situations such as that at St. Lawrence, since they contained a form of compulsory arbitration and could facilitate third-party intervention.

Though now armed with ample legislative power to do so, Woods still refused to appoint an inquiry into the St. Lawrence dispute. However, further developments forced his hand. Because of its importance to the steel and aluminum industries, fluorspar was crucial to the war effort, and the St. Lawrence mines were the main supplier of fluorspar to Canadian consumers. Two weeks into the strike by St. Lawrence Corporation workers, the Secretary of State for External Affairs in Ottawa began to press Woods for a resolution to the St. Lawrence dispute.[36] Shortly thereafter, workers at Newfluor, who had stayed on the job throughout previous disputes, walked out to demand a wage increase and to support their fellow members employed at the St. Lawrence Corporation (*Evening Telegram* November 7, 1941).

The work stoppage at Newfluor posed a further threat to the fluorspar supply and placed Woods under increased pressure from government and corporate officials in Canada. The Canadian Secretary of State reminded Woods that there was no Canadian source of fluorspar and that "continued supplies of Fluorspar from Newfoundland are of utmost importance for Canadian steel and aluminum industries."[37] The president of Dosco, the St. Lawrence Corporation's main customer, told Woods that it was "absolutely essential" that the supply from St. Lawrence be maintained.[38] The union reminded Woods that workers were aware of the importance of fluorspar to the war effort and of the far-reaching implications of the labour dispute.[39] In these circumstances, Woods had little choice but to accede to the union's demands for an inquiry. He informed the union that the government would establish a Trade Dispute Board, and in compliance with the regulations the men went back to work.[40]

"Miscellaneous Matters": The Trade Dispute Board Settlement

The Trade Dispute Board arrived in St. Lawrence in January 1942. The composition of the Board, particularly the choice of union representative, and the terms of reference may have had something to do with the eventual outcome. The government-appointed union representative was W.J. Walsh, former Minister of Agriculture and Mines in the last pre-Commission administration. Thomas J. Lefeuvre, a businessman and former politician from the St. Lawrence area, represented the employers, while Professor A.M. Fraser of Memorial University College was designated the third, impartial member. Despite the many complaints raised by the union in the time leading up to the inquiry, the terms of reference did not include health and safety — only the employment of non-union men, union recognition, and wages.

Over the course of the inquiry, the Board would examine sixty-five written submissions and hear twenty-one witnesses, including Turpin, Poynter, and twelve workers (*Evening Telegram* December 6, 1941). Poynter's testimony regarding his company's financial situation was taken "in private at the Manager's office" (Newfoundland 1942, 3–4, 10). While not officially subject to the Board's inquiry, Newfluor had agreed to abide by the Board's rulings.

The Board gave qualified support to the union's demand for recognition. It ruled that since there were just eight non-union men on the payroll, the St. Lawrence Corporation should recognize the SLWPU as the sole bargaining agent for its employees, but that any non-union employee on the payroll as of December 1, 1941, should not be required to join the union (Newfoundland 1942, 30). The Board also ruled favourably on the union's demand for a wage increase to keep pace with wartime inflation, ordering the St. Lawrence Corporation to raise its base wage and pay a cost-of-living increase as of March 1942 (Newfoundland 1942, 30-40).

Workers and the union president insisted on bringing concerns over health hazards to the Board's attention, despite the fact that they were not included in the official terms of reference. These included "foul air," inadequate ventilation, and the dust created by dry-drilling, which workers believed was "injurious to the eyes and lungs." Discussion of these issues was relegated to a section entitled "Miscellaneous Matters" in the Board's final report.

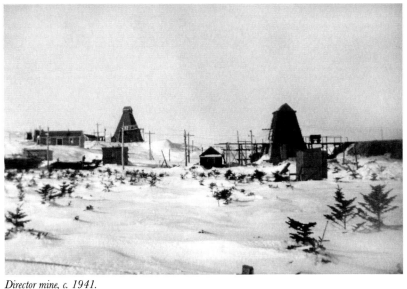

Director mine, c. 1941.

The report downplayed complaints of foul air, stating that "in the most efficiently operated mines in the world, there is certain to be foul air at times" (Newfoundland 1942, 48). The report also pointed out that on a recent tour of one St. Lawrence Corporation mine, Board members had not noticed any foul air. What the report did not point out was that during that tour, many sections of this mine were still flooded and inaccessible because of the recent work stoppage, while the St. Lawrence Corporation's other two main mines were completely flooded and could not be entered at all (Newfoundland 1942, 6–7). The tour was thus far from sufficient to convey an accurate sense of normal working conditions. As for the use of dry drills,

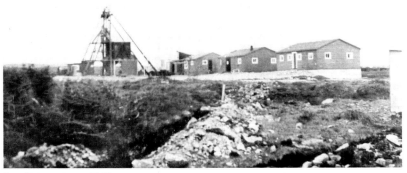

Iron Springs mine, c. 1942.

Poynter denied to the Board that the dry drill was used in the St. Lawrence Corporation mines, but the Board reported that it was in fact employed and urged that "this type of hammer be no longer used except in those parts of the mine where ground water renders it innocuous" (Newfoundland 1942, 48–49).

Turpin and the workers also complained of the lack of medical services. A doctor had come to St. Lawrence early in 1941, with the mining companies and the employees each paying a portion of the expenses (the employees paid fifty cents monthly), but had left in December of that year. Miners had donated labour to the partial construction of a rough building that might be used as a hospital, but there was no money for finishing or equipping it. Several workers and the union president expressed concern about the lack of medical facilities since they wanted some way of testing their belief that dust and inadequate ventilation were damaging workers' health and that "due to the conditions they would die eventually with lung trouble."[41] The union urged the Board to make some provision to conduct chest x-rays on the miners until a more permanent arrangement could be established (Newfoundland 1942, 50).

The Board's report conceded that the community was sorely lacking in medical services and urged the companies and the union to cooperate in approaching the Department of Public Health and Welfare for advice in trying to obtain a doctor for the community. There was no suggestion, however, that the government provide anything other than advice (Newfoundland 1942, 49–51). As for the request for chest x-rays, the Board responded: "We are not competent to pronounce as to the necessity for such an examination, but we desire to place the Union's wishes on record, as they were expressed very strongly" (Newfoundland 1942, 51).

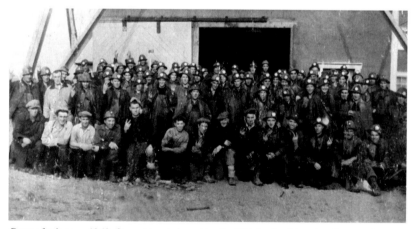

Group of miners, c. 1943. Some appear to be making the "V" sign for victory, in reference to the war.

Ongoing Hazards and Industry Decline, 1942–45

In the immediate aftermath of the Trade Dispute Board settlement, an event occurred that would have a lasting effect upon the community. On the night of February 17, 1942, two U.S. naval ships went aground near the town — the destroyer Truxton near the Iron Springs mine and the supply ship Pollux just west of there. A Truxton crewmember made it to the Iron Springs mine, and workers, soon joined by others from the community, began the arduous task of pulling survivors from the icy, oil-soaked waters. The people of the town of Lawn undertook a similar effort at the Pollux wreck, which had been spotted by a hunter from that community. About 200 sailors died, but 168 were rescued and taken into homes in St. Lawrence and Lawn to be nursed back to health. In addition to occupying an important place in the history of the area and the consciousness of the people, the rescue effort would result in the U.S. government funding construction of a hospital at St. Lawrence more than a decade later (Brown 1979).

Meanwhile, the union continued to pressure the mining companies and the government to help provide medical services for the community.[42] That services were inadequate was made clear by an incident in August 1942, when a worker was killed by a 120-foot fall down the Iron Springs shaft. Workers retrieved his body in an ore bucket and laid it on a lunchroom table. It was examined by a member of the mine's supervisory staff, who pronounced the man dead.[43] Even some government employees were openly appalled at the state of medical services in the community. In his report on the accident, the Ranger expressed his dismay at "the lack of medical aid in this place… [with]… an operation of the nature and scale of the one now being carried on here." The District Magistrate supported the Ranger's view, suggesting that the medical situation in St. Lawrence was "probably without parallel in the whole of the British Commonwealth."[44] He urged the government to pass a law requiring the establishment and maintenance of adequate medical services in St. Lawrence.

The union also continued to complain about health hazards. About six months after the Trade Dispute Board settlement, the union again complained to the government about inadequate ventilation and heavy dust in the mines. Significantly, these complaints included Newfluor's Director mine, which had recently moved from the developmental phase to production. The complaints were again dismissed, with the Governor remarking that there was "no reason for apprehension."[45]

While continuing to disregard specific health concerns, the government did continue to bring in mine inspectors from Ontario periodically. An inspection carried out by D.G. Sinclair in October 1943 found that many shafts at St. Lawrence were now up to 400 feet deep, with over 1,000 feet of drifting carried out in some places. Such changes had no doubt increased the need for ventilation, since workers at the far end of a drift were now up to 1,400 feet from the nearest source of air, and as Sinclair pointed out, the only openings from the underground to the surface were the main shafts.[46] Sinclair also reiterated the need to overhaul the legislation and upgrade the inspection service, noting that even the outdated provisions of the 1908 Act were not being complied with or enforced. He suggested that in adopting a new code, the government follow the process that had been used in Ontario regulations and give industry and labour the opportunity to contribute.[47] Woods suggested that a draft code be circulated to the management of Newfoundland's mines, but not to the unions as Sinclair recommended. Woods also observed that drafting new regulations might shield the government from possible criticism "if circumstances leading to a disaster are shown even faintly to have been such that lack of control by the State has any bearing in the case."[48] However, not even such pragmatic considerations were sufficient to invoke action, and no legislative changes were forthcoming.

While the government maintained the status quo with respect to its role in addressing health and safety concerns, a notable change was taking place in the sphere of labour relations: the inclusion of health and safety provisions in collective agreements that the SLWPU eventually signed with both companies to supplant the Trade Dispute Board settlement. In October 1942, the SLWPU and Newfluor entered into a collective agreement that essentially embodied the same terms as the settlement. The union renegotiated the agreement with Newfluor in May 1944 and at the same time signed its first agreement with the St. Lawrence Corporation. In addition to some moderate wage increases, both agreements contained clauses dealing with health and safety and with medical services. The agreements called for the appointment of one or more workers to be "responsible at all times that the mines were safe for the men to work." Both employers also pledged to help secure a doctor on a more permanent basis and to contribute a share of the cost, provided the remainder was funded by other sources.[49] Two physicians came to St. Lawrence under this arrangement, but neither stayed more than a few months.

The union may have continued to push for improvements in health and safety and other matters, but an industry decline beginning in 1944 hampered its efforts. By the end of 1943, the mines had a combined workforce of about 700, but early the following year a decline in production at the Arvida plant led to reduced demand for fluorspar and Newfluor began laying off workers. By March 1944, its workforce was down to less than 200, compared to a high of 350 in 1943.[50] By January 1945, Newfluor employed just eighty workers, and by the end of the war operations had ceased entirely.[51]

The St. Lawrence Corporation maintained a high level of production throughout much of 1944, owing largely to an agreement with the War

Production Board of the U.S. Department of National Defence, under which the company supplied fluorspar in exchange for financial assistance to expand the St. Lawrence operation (Hiley 1945 5–13). Initially the St. Lawrence Corporation absorbed some of the displaced workers from Newfluor, but in the fall of 1944 that company also began curtailing production, shutting down two of its four mines.[52] The decline continued through 1945, and by the end of that year the St. Lawrence Corporation employed just 150 men.[53]

Industry decline at the end of the war had a direct impact on the labour relations environment. One observer remarked in 1944 that "the fact that jobs are not so plentiful as they were last year, is one of the main reasons why there is not likely to be so much trouble from now on."[54] In fact, the union was losing ground on some of the few gains it had made to date, including a 10 percent reduction in wages in 1945.[55]

An increase in unemployment and requests for relief during 1945 highlight the effects of a decade of mining upon the economy and the labour force. Clearly, people had little to fall back on as the mining industry declined. Some had returned to fishing, but the number of boats and fishing premises had declined since 1935 and fishing was clearly less prominent in St. Lawrence than in other nearby communities (Newfoundland Department of Public Health and Welfare 1946).

It is also apparent that by 1945 the social and economic divisions that would eventually become a source of tension and conflict were beginning to emerge. While the vast majority of rank and file workers were native to St. Lawrence or nearby communities, much of the supervisory staff had been recruited from outside the area. Warren Smith, Newfluor's mine manager, was from the United States, while Newfluor Mining Captain Murdock Judson was from Canada. These occupational distinctions were of course reflected in income levels; for example, St. Lawrence Corporation manager Donald Poynter reported an annual salary of $6,000 per year in 1945, roughly five times the income of a St. Lawrence miner (Newfoundland Department of Public Health and Welfare 1946).

Public Relief applications also point to the issues of health and health services. Regarding unemployed miners seeking relief, the local Relieving Officer made the suggestive but unexplained remark: "In some cases it is questionable that some applicants are really able-bodied but there is no way for them to secure medical certificates without travelling to Grand Bank or Burin for examination."[56] The lack of reliable records — a factor compounded by absence of medical facilities — makes it difficult to determine the exact impact that health hazards may have had at this stage, but it would soon become apparent that for their $100 a month many miners were giving not only their labour but their health and, eventually, their lives.

Notes

1. Resume of negotiations for Newfoundland fluorspar properties, 31 July 1940, Archival Collection of the Aluminum Company of Canada (hereafter AA).
2. E.J. Lavino, E.J. Lavino and Company, to Warren Smith, Manager, American-Newfoundland Fluorspar, St. Lawrence, 28 March 1939, AA.
3. Report made by Magistrate Short on the subject of a dispute between the St. Lawrence Corporation of Newfoundland Ltd., and the St. Lawrence Miners and Labourers Protective Union, 23 May 1940, GN38, S5-4-1, File 5, PANL.
4. Report made by Magistrate Short on the subject of a dispute between the St. Lawrence Corporation of Newfoundland Ltd., and the St. Lawrence Miners and Labourers Protective Union, 23 May 1940, GN38, S5-4-1, File 5, PANL.
5. Report made by Magistrate Short on the subject of a dispute between the St. Lawrence Corporation of Newfoundland Ltd., and the St. Lawrence Miners and Labourers Protective Union, 23 May 1940, GN38, S5-4-1, File 5, PANL.
6. Report made by Magistrate Short on the subject of a dispute between the St. Lawrence Corporation of Newfoundland Ltd., and the St. Lawrence Miners and Labourers Protective Union, 23 May 1940, GN38, S5-4-1, File 5, PANL.
7. Report made by Magistrate Short on the subject of a dispute between the St. Lawrence Corporation of Newfoundland Ltd., and the St. Lawrence Miners and Labourers Protective Union, 23 May 1940, GN38, S5-4-1, File 5, PANL.
8. Report made by Magistrate Short on the subject of a dispute between the St. Lawrence Corporation of Newfoundland Ltd., and the St. Lawrence Miners and Labourers Protective Union, 23 May 1940, GN38, S5-4-1, File 5, PANL.
9. Report made by Magistrate Short on the subject of a dispute between the St. Lawrence Corporation of Newfoundland Ltd., and the St. Lawrence Miners and Labourers Protective Union, 23 May 1940, GN38, S5-4-1, File 5, PANL.
10. Report made by Magistrate Short on the subject of a dispute between the St. Lawrence Corporation of Newfoundland Ltd., and the St. Lawrence Miners and Labourers Protective Union, 23 May 1940, GN38, S5-4-1, File 5, PANL.
11. Inspection Report on the Mining Operations in Newfoundland, 1940, DME.
12. Interview with Aloysius Turpin, Montreal, 24 June 1967, Memorial University of Newfoundland Folklore and Language Archive (hereafter MUNFLA), Collection 84-224, Tapes C7239, 7240, 7241.
13. Interview with Aloysius Turpin, MUNFLA.
14. Turpin to Donald Poynter, Manager, St. Lawrence Corporation of Newfoundland, 5 May 1941 MM.
15. Poynter to Turpin, 5 May 1941 MM.
16. W.S Smith, Manager, Newfoundland Fluorspar Limited, to Aloysius Turpin, President, SLWPU, 24 April 194, MM.
17. Poynter to Turpin, 5 May 1941 MM.
18. P.J. Lewis to Wilfrid Woods, Commissioner of Public Utilities, 27 May 1941, GN38, S5-4-1, File 6, PANL.
19. Lewis to Woods, 27 May 1941, GN38, S5-4-1, File 6, PANL.
20. Memorandum for the Commission of Government from Sir Wilfrid Woods, 17 January 1941, GN38, S4-2-5, File 2, PANL.
21. Lewis to Turpin, 27 May 1941, MM.

22. Woods to Lewis, 30 May 1941; and MM, Lewis to Woods, 14 July 1941, GN38, S5-4-1, File 6, PANL.
23. Woods to Lewis, 15 July 1941, GN38, S5-4-1, File 6, PANL.
24. Turpin to Woods, and Lewis to Woods, 17 July 1941, GN 38, S5-4-1, File 6, PANL.
25. Walter Seibert, President, St. Lawrence Corporation of Newfoundland, to Woods, 22 July 1941, GN 38, S5-4-1, File 6, PANL.
26. Seibert to Woods, 22 July 1941, GN 38, S5-4-1, File 6, PANL.
27. Woods to Lewis, 24 July 1941, GN38, S5-4-1, File 6, PANL.
28. Lewis to Turpin, 20 August 1941, MM; and Lewis to Woods, 4 September 1941, GN38, S5-4-1, File 6, PANL.
29. Memorandum from Sir Wilfrid Woods for the Commission of Government, 5 September 1941, GN38, S5-4-1, File 6, PANL.
30. Memorandum from Sir Wilfrid Woods for the Commission of Government, 5 September 1941, GN38, S5-4-1, File 6, PANL.
31. Memorandum from Sir Wilfrid Woods for the Commission of Government, 25 October 1941, GN38, S5-4-1, File 5, PANL.
32. Poynter to Woods, 28 October 1941, GN38, S5-6-1, File 5, PANL.
33. Lewis to Woods, 1 November 1941, GN38, S5-6-1, File 5, PANL.
34. Defence (Control and Conditions of Employment and Disputes Settlement) Regulations, 23 October 1941 (St. John's 1941).
35. Defence (Control and Conditions of Employment and Disputes Settlement) Regulations, 23 October 1941 (St. John's 1941).
36. C.J. Burchell, High Commissioner for Canada in St. John's, to Woods, containing a telegram from Burchell to Secretary of State for External Affairs, Ottawa, 3 November 1941, GN38, S5-4-1, File 5, PANL.
37. Burchell to Woods, containing a copy of a telegram from the Secretary of State for External Affairs, Ottawa, 8 November 1941, GN38, S5-4-1, File 5, PANL.
38. A. Cross, President, Dominion Steel and Coal Corporation, Montreal, to the Woods, 7 December 1941, GN 38 S5-4-1, File 5, PANL.
39. Lewis to Woods, 1 November 1941, GN38, S5-6-1, File 5, PANL.
40. Lewis to Woods, 10 November 1941, PANL, GN38, S5-4-1, File 5; Woods to Lewis, 10 November 1941, GN38, S5-4-1, File 5, PANL; and Lewis to Turpin, 17 November 1941, MM.
41. Interview with Aloysius Turpin, MUNFLA.
42. Governor Humphrey Walwyn to Clement B. Atlee Secretary of State for Dominion Affairs, 25 August 1942, GN38, S5-4-1, File 5, PANL.
43. "Report on Fatal Accident, St. Lawrence, 19 August 1942," GN 4/1/D, G/100/1, PANL.
44. "Report on Fatal Accident, St. Lawrence, 19 August 1942," GN 4/1/D, G/100/1, PANL.
45. Governor Humphrey Walwyn to Clement B. Atlee, Secretary of State for Dominion Affairs, 25 August 1942, GN38, S5-4-1, File 5, PANL.
46. Report of Dr. D.G. Sinclair, Assistant Deputy Minister of Mines for Ontario on Mining Operations in Newfoundland, 29 January 1944, GN38, S5-1-3 (PU 17-44), PANL.

47. D.G. Sinclair to Claude K. Howse, 27 October 1943, GN38, S5-1-3 (PU 17-44), PANL.

48. Memorandum from Sir Wilfrid Woods, circulated to the Commission of Government, 29 January 1944, GN38, S5-1-3 (PU 17-44), PANL.

49. Agreement between St. Lawrence Corporation of Newfoundland Limited and St. Lawrence Workers' Protective Union, 10 May 1944; and MM; and Agreement between Newfoundland Fluorspar Limited and St. Lawrence Workers' Protective Union, 12 May 1944, MM.

50. List of men on Newfluor payroll, 1943 and 1944, MM.

51. Report of the Ranger, St. Lawrence Detachment, for July to December, 1945, GN38, S2-5, PANL.

52. Report of the Ranger, St. Lawrence Detachment, for September 1944, GN38, S2-5-2; and Report of the Ranger, St. Lawrence Detachment, for October 1944, GN38, S2-5-2, PANL.

53. Report of the Ranger, St. Lawrence Detachment, for July to December 1945, GN38, S2-5-2, PANL.

54. Report of the Ranger, St. Lawrence Detachment, for January to June 1944, GN38, S2-5-2, PANL.

55. Report of the Ranger, St. Lawrence Detachment, for July to December 1945, GN38, S2-5-2, PANL.

56. Report of the Ranger, St. Lawrence Detachment, for July to December, 1945, GN38, S2-5-2, PANL.

Chapter Three

INDUSTRY REVIVAL, INCREASING HAZARDS AND THE RECOGNITION OF SILICOSIS, 1946–1956

The Post-War Revival

After the curtailment of operations during the mid-1940s, the industry revived with a surge in the demand for fluorspar late in the decade. Advances in aluminum production fostered by the war made aluminum a popular product with public and industrial consumers. This increased demand led to Alcan's becoming one of the largest producers of raw aluminum in the world and prompted it to open a new, expanded plant at Arvida in 1948. The outbreak of the Korean War in 1950 furthered industry expansion as American firms such as Alcoa and Kaiser Aluminum entered into contracts with Alcan for the supply of raw aluminum, which these companies in turn used to fulfill supply contracts with the U.S. government.

To help supply the expanded Arvida plant, Newfluor revived the Director mine, and by 1948 production there had rebounded to equal the record level of 1943.[1] Newfluor also began a second shaft on the Director vein, which was at 400 feet by 1952 and 550 feet by 1955,[2] and it constructed a new mill, similar to the St. Lawrence Corporation's, which went into production in January 1951.[3]

The St. Lawrence Corporation continued to operate on a reduced basis during the years immediately following the war, but despite this reduction, the owners established a processing plant in Wilmington, Delaware, under the name St. Lawrence Fluorspar of Delaware, to treat the St. Lawrence product before sending it on to American consumers (Peat, Marwick, Mitchell and Company 1950). Like Newfluor, the St. Lawrence Corporation saw an opportunity to expand production and take advantage of the increase in American and Canadian demand for fluorspar.[4] However, its president, Seibert, claimed that to do so the company required an infusion of $250,000 in capital, and he turned to the Newfoundland government for help in securing a loan.

Seibert was now dealing with the government of the newly established Province of Newfoundland. Newfoundland's political status had changed in response to the economic recovery that had accompanied the war. In a plebiscite held on July 21, 1948, just over 52 percent of the voters supported confederation with Canada while the remainder supported a return to Responsible Government. Newfoundland thus became the tenth province of Canada on March 31, 1949, and the victorious confederates, led by Joseph Smallwood under the Liberal Party banner, became the provincial government in May 1949 (Noel 1971, 248–62; Neary 1988, 313–45). Smallwood's Liberals would hold power until the early 1970s.

Shortly after the government took office, Seibert informed Smallwood that should the company be unable to secure credit, it would be forced to shut down the St. Lawrence operation.[5] An audit ordered by the government reveals little of the St. Lawrence Corporation's financial status, since for most purposes the audit treats the St. Lawrence Corporation and the Delaware company as a single entity. It is clear, however, that after showing losses during 1946–47, the combined companies began reporting profits in 1948. The St. Lawrence Corporation itself reported profits each year from 1946 to 1949. The audit also showed that a "Staff House" recently constructed as the manager's residence and a social club for staff members cost $25,000 — more than a hundred times the amount spent on a so-called "ventilation system" for the Iron Springs mine. (The average value of a St. Lawrence miner's house at that time was about $1,500.) Ultimately, the auditing firm concluded that though it appeared risky from the strictly financial viewpoint, the government should guarantee the loan given the importance of the industry to the community and to the province (Peat, Marwick, Mitchell and Company 1950, Schedule 7).

Having thus secured financial assistance, the St. Lawrence Corporation expanded operations and stepped up production. By 1952, the Iron Springs shaft was down to 780 feet and several thousand additional feet of drifting had been carried out. The company also reactivated several other sites that had been shut down for several years and developed some new ones. At the Blue Beach mine, the shaft was extended from 130 to 230 feet, and a second shaft was sunk to the 185-foot level. The Lord and Lady Gulch site, which had been abandoned in 1937, was also revived in the early 1950s, and the St. Lawrence Corporation sank a small shaft on another vein known as the Grassy Gulch.[7] In 1955 the Iron Springs mine, which continued to be the St. Lawrence Corporation's primary producer, was extended to the 890-foot level and further drifting carried out, while expansion continued at the Blue Beach mine and other sites.[7]

The St. Lawrence Corporation benefitted further from the increased demand for fluorspar created by the U.S. entry into the Korean War. In 1952, it entered into a contract with the United States Defense Materials Procurement Agency to supply 150,000 tons of acid-grade fluorspar over the next four years. As part of this agreement, the United States government advanced the St. Lawrence Corporation $1,250,000 to upgrade and expand its processing facilities at both St. Lawrence and Wilmington. The St. Lawrence Corporation was to repay some of this money with the fluorspar itself, as a portion of each ton shipped. The expansion program included upgrading the St. Lawrence mill to produce high-grade ore to be shipped to the Wilmington plant for further refining. The Wilmington plant thus became the main destination for the St. Lawrence Corporation's product, though small amounts of metallurgical grade ore were sometimes shipped directly to steel plants in both the U.S. and Canada.[8]

This industry growth was reflected in both employment and population levels: by 1956 over 500 people were directly employed in the mining industry and the town's population had increased to more than 1,800 — from about 1,400 in 1949 (Newfoundland Department of Mines and Resources 1957; Newfoundland Department of Finance 1970, Volume 1, Table A-1, Table A-17). The vast majority of workers continued to be residents of St. Lawrence, but the mines drew many from neighbouring communities as well. Some settled in St. Lawrence, while others commuted daily, found lodging in private homes, or lived in crude bunkhouses constructed near the mines.[9]

The resurgence of the mining industry in the 1950s again altered the composition of the community's labour force. After many had eventually returned to fishing during the postwar slump, in 1955 only three people in St. Lawrence reported fishing as their primary occupation (Newfoundland Chief Electoral Officer 1956, 95–115). The industry expansion and increase in population led to a growth in retail, service, and other industries in the community. New stores, bars, and other small businesses were opened, one effect being to draw more women into the paid workforce (Newfoundland Chief Electoral Officer 1956, 95–115).

An Interlude in Union Leadership and Status

In 1946, James Cusick, a forty-seven-year-old veteran miner who had started as a driller in 1935 and risen to become driller foreman by 1945, challenged Turpin for the presidency of the union. Why the majority of members supported Cusick's bid is unclear, but may reflect the fact that the latest contract negotiated under Turpin (late in 1945) had included a 10 percent cut in pay.[10]

In 1949, Cusick was approached by a representative of the American Federation of Labour–Trades and Labor Congress (AFL-TLC) about having the SLWPU affiliate with that organization. Continental organizations such as the AFL-TLC and the Canadian Congress of Labour–Congress of Industrial Organizations (CCL-CIO) had been seeking affiliates among Newfoundland unions throughout the late 1940s, part of a general trend paralleling Newfoundland's political integration into Canada.[11] Cusick later recalled that he supported affiliation because he believed that an independent union lacked the power to negotiate successfully and that remaining independent played into the hands of employers. According to Cusick, SLWPU members voted unanimously to affiliate with the AFL-CIO.[12] In May 1949, the SLWPU became Federal Labour Union (FLU) 24530. FLUs were directly affiliated with the AFL, as opposed to coming under the AFL by way of membership in an AFL-affiliated international body (Zieger 1977, 1–38; Taft 1959, 98–108).

During the seven years of affiliation with the AFL-CIO, there were brief disputes over such matters as wages and benefits, but the labour relations environment was generally quiet. Agreements negotiated with both companies during the first half of the 1950s contained wage increases and improvements in such areas as annual vacations. To Cusick, these gains were an indication of the benefits of affiliation, and he later claimed that without the support and expertise of the parent organization, the union never could have made such progress during this time.[13] Indeed, financial information the AFL-CIO staff provided on both companies was used by Cusick to support the union's demands; the fact that profits for the St. Lawrence Corporation increased substantially from 1949 to 1951,[14] for instance, countered the Corporation's continuing claims that it was cash-poor and could not afford wage increases or other concessions.[15]

When Cusick resigned in 1954 to take a job elsewhere, Turpin seized the chance to regain the presidency. Turpin made it clear from the outset that he had not changed his mind about affiliation and that he wanted the union to "get out from under" the AFL-TLC as soon as possible. This desire seems to have derived in part from Turpin's animosity towards the AFL-TLC's Newfoundland representative.[16] Early in March 1956, Turpin got the support of the membership to break the affiliation, partly by generating resentment over an AFL-TLC request for the union's per capita fees.[17]

The Fiction and Fact of Working Conditions

A striking feature of the period of Cusick's presidency and affiliation with the AFL-TLC was the relative lack of attention paid to health and safety issues. Cusick did raise such concerns on occasion, such as during negotiations with the St. Lawrence Corporation in 1953, when he criticized the lack of sanitary facilities in the workplace and pointed out that a blower system purchased for Iron Springs mine had never been installed. On the whole, though, workplace hazards seem not to have been prominent issues for the union during this period. This may simply have reflected Cusick's style and priorities, or it may have been a more structural matter related to affiliation with an organization that had little direct knowledge of the workplace hazards at St. Lawrence and of measures to address them.

What is clear is that there was no shortage of hazards. Having not yet established its own inspectorate, in 1949 the provincial government brought in another mines inspector, A.V. Corlett, from Ontario. Corlett's comments are revealing. His observation that a "raise" (a vertical opening) was being created from the 250-foot level to the surface at Director mine, a step management stated would eventually provide ventilation, raises questions about what if any ventilation existed there at the time. As for the St. Lawrence Corporation mines, Corlett was appalled at the hoisting system in use at Blue Beach, which he described as "completely unsuitable for mine hoisting work and not be acceptable under any modern code of mine-hoisting requirements." In what had become a familiar move, the St. Lawrence Corporation had temporarily suspended operations at Iron Springs during the inspection so Corlett did not visit the underground there. However, he was assured by the Mine Captain that in response to suggestions arising from previous inspections, the company was also creating raises for emergency exits and for ventilation. Corlett noted that with the 1908 Code hopelessly out of date and the inspection service completely inadequate, operators had essentially been left to govern themselves as they pleased, and he urged the government to move quickly in updating protective measures.[18]

Corlett repeated these suggestions after another visit in 1950. During this inspection, the St. Lawrence Corporation again scaled back operations, reportedly because of a power shortage. Even so, Corlett noted that due to an accidental breakthrough from a stope on the 450-foot level into the shaft, there was much better airflow in one level of the Iron Springs mine than on others where no ventilation existed. Corlett recommended that raises be created to provide exists and ventilation on all levels.[19]

On what would be his final visit, in 1951, Corlett noted that two new raises had been driven to the surface at the Director mine, one of which was being used for ventilation and the other as an escape way. He was told, however, that this was a temporary arrangement: eventually these openings would be used as channels for pumping water and as escape exits. This contradicted what Corlett had been told in 1949 — that one of these raises was intended to be used for ventilation. Corlett noted that there were still no mine plans for any of the St. Lawrence Corporation mines, no ventilation raises at the Iron Springs mine, and serious problems with the hoisting equipment despite repeated requests to bring it up to standard. Corlett also pointed out that the St. Lawrence Corporation continued to have the highest accident rate in Newfoundland mines and that Newfluor's rate was the second highest.[20]

While Corlett conducted inspections from 1949 to 1951, the provincial government was drafting new legislation, The Act Respecting the Safety of Workmen in Mines, which took effect in 1951. The legislation covered most standard concerns, including hoisting, flooding, fires, explosives, and electrical installations. It also stated that the ventilation in every mine should be such that the air in all areas "is free from dangerous amounts of noxious impurities, including dust, and contains sufficient oxygen to ensure the health of anyone employed in the mine." The legislation required that if such conditions could not be achieved by natural ventilation, "means for mechanical ventilation shall be provided and kept in operation." Other sections of the Act required operators to supply workers with masks approved by the chief inspector to protect them from "dust, gas, and irritating and dangerous fumes" (Newfoundland 1952).

The provisions of the Newfoundland legislation differed from those in other Canadian jurisdictions in a number of important ways. For example, while inspectors brought in from Ontario had encouraged Newfoundland mine operators since the 1930s to emulate Ontario standards, the Newfoundland provisions diverged in at least one crucial area: Ontario had stringent requirements for medical examination of workers in designated "dust exposure occupations," which included all underground miners. Those applying for employment in these occupations had to be deemed free from all diseases of the respiratory system and examined annually to maintain their eligibility. Newfoundland's Act also differed from Ontario's in requiring neither a supply of water to suppress dust underground nor detailed ventilation plans for underground areas (Ontario 1949). The Nova Scotia law also required that water be supplied to suppress dust and added that no person was to work in any area containing "dust, fumes or smoke perceptible to the senses," while both Ontario and Nova Scotia required wet drills (Ontario 1949; Nova Scotia 1952). Significantly, while the Ontario and Nova Scotia legislation contained a requirement to suppress dust, neither contained the Newfoundland requirement for wearing masks. It is as if those who drafted the Newfoundland code were resigned to the presence of dust in the mines and, rather than attempt to reduce or eliminate it, simply adopted measures to cope with it.

Despite these limitations, the new legislation was a vast improvement on what had existed previously. Whether it would improve health and safety, however, depended on how it was administered. One of the factors that no doubt came into play in this regard was the Smallwood government's emphasis on the potential for mining and other land-based resources to ensure the province's future prosperity. Under Smallwood's mantra of "Develop, Develop, Develop," one of the provincial government's first moves after coming to power was to grant extensive rights to private interests that planned to explore and develop resources on the island and in Labrador. During this period, the vast iron ore deposits in western Labrador were the subject of a great deal of interest, and by the early 1960s the Iron Ore Company of Canada had developed major mining operations at two of these sites, which would become Wabush and Labrador City. The international giant Johns-Manville Company had begun mining an asbestos deposit at Baie Verte on the island's northeast coast in 1955, an operation that would ultimately claim many lives through asbestosis and other work-related diseases.

Where health and safety fit into the new government's priorities was reflected in the words of the first Chief Inspector of Mines, Fred Gover. Shortly after his appointment, Gover remarked that while the primary purpose of the legislation was to protect workers, "so much importance" was being placed on this purpose that "we are apt to forget that a Regulations of Mines Act is the only instrument which society employs to ensure that none of nature's mineral gifts will be plundered or wasted in the process of extraction."[21] In other words, the Chief Inspector believed that a large part of his role was to address the imbalance that had resulted from placing too much emphasis on health and safety and not enough on developing the industry.

The inspectorate's approach to addressing health and safety concerns was also reflected in its early reports, from which one would assume there was little cause for concern. The inspectorate's report for 1953, for example, noted that as a result of tests carried out that year, "more is known about air conditions underground than was known since mining first began in Newfoundland [and] the consequence of this is a feeling of confidence throughout the industry that our mines are safe and healthy places to work" (Newfoundland Department of Mines and Resources 1954, 65–67). There was no indication, however, of what exactly the 1953 survey had revealed about air conditions. The report also noted that mines across the province had been tested for dust and that mine managers had been given the results of the survey with the "expectation" that they would take "such action as appeared necessary" (Newfoundland Department of Mines and Resources 1954, 65–67). The same report stated that in Newfoundland mines, "the presence of a good supply of oxygen is also ensured by constant examination and ventilation." Significantly, the 1953 report included the Mines Branch's intention to abdicate its responsibility for air testing, which was to be handed over to mine operators, and to retain responsibility only for analysis. The Branch conceded, however, that it was not properly equipped even for this limited task. It had to send the samples to Quebec for analysis, which often resulted in breakage and the settling of dust in the sample flasks during shipment (Newfoundland Department of Mines and Resources 1954, 76–79).

The report for 1954 continued the trend of vague assurances and supposedly positive developments. It referred to unspecified steps being taken to reduce "potential gas and dust hazards" in Newfoundland mines and praised the cooperation of mine operators in these efforts (Newfoundland Department of Mines and Resources 1955, 98–100). It also noted that there had been "no adverse reports" of health effects associated with diesel-powered tram cars recently introduced at Director mine (Newfoundland Department of Mines and Resources 1955, 127–29). Overall, the inspection reports from this period appear to have functioned largely as a public relations device, both to create the impression of safe and healthy conditions and to stress how technological advances (such as the diesel trams) had improved efficiency and productivity in the industry.

Those who worked in the St. Lawrence mines during the 1950s tell a very different story. Jerome Spearns, a thoughtful and soft-spoken man who speaks fondly of the many former co-workers he has watched die over the years, started work as a driller at Iron Springs in 1951 and described conditions there during the 1950s:

> Unbelievable. I was gassed every day I was there. I'd have to come up out of the mine half the time. Not only me. There was as high as twenty of us had to come up at a time. All they used to say was, can't go down there, too much gas down there. You'd go down and you'd start to get a headache, real bad, as soon as you'd get there, sometimes you wouldn't be able to stay a half hour. But if you got the water hose going and got the air, then you kind of cleared it up, and you'd manage to go back and spend a shift, but you'd have this headache all day.[22]

Spearns recalled that dry-drilling still went on in the 1950s when no water was available or when there was insufficient water pressure to reach working areas. He also noted the problem of fumes from the diesel fuel that was burned in some equipment, combined with the complete absence of ventilation in many working areas. Men were reluctant to complain about these conditions, Spearns said, for fear of losing their jobs.[23]

Adrian Slaney went to work with the St. Lawrence Corporation in 1952. An articulate and insightful man who died of cancer in 2002, he also described a situation very different from that depicted in the official reports. Slaney recalled that there was simply no ventilation in the Iron Springs mine and the air grew thinner as workers moved away from the shaft and out into the drifts:

> When you got away from the shaft, you could forget about lighting a cigarette.... If you heard the elevator rushing down the shaft and you wanted a smoke bad enough you ran back to the shaft because she'd push a certain quantity of air down ahead of her, so you had to hurry up and light the match and then you'd keep puffing the cigarette to keep it lit.... Over a period of time the boys devised their own ways of getting air.... Far out in the tunnel where there was no such thing as air, they would open a valve every now and then [from air supply lines to drills and other equipment] and breathe in that way, and the boys up in the stope would unscrew the hose from the

end of the drill and get air and then hook it up again.[24]

Adrian Slaney recalled that workers were often overcome and would "just collapse on the track… just pass out." When that happened, they would be brought to the surface and laid out on the dryhouse floor:

> I counted twenty-one men one time just laying there…. The surface air would bring them around but they'd have this terrible splitting headache. [The Mine Captain] would give them an aspirin and a drink of water, and they'd dress up and go down again…. They'd work and pass out again sometimes.[25]

Slaney also described dust so thick that you could not see a person working next to you and the light from his hat would be a dim orange glow. "Nobody wore masks," he stated, "at the St. Lawrence Corporation or at Alcan, underground, in the lab or in the mill." One of the things that made conditions bad at smaller sites the St. Lawrence Corporation developed throughout the 1950s, according to Slaney, was the practice of using equipment (such as dry drills) that had been worn out and abandoned at larger operations.[26]

Conditions at Newfluor's Director mine were reportedly not much better. Richard "Bud" Loder is a burly man who went to work at Director in 1953, when he was just seventeen years old. While not legally old enough to work underground at the time, he recalled with a chuckle that he was "big enough." Regarding Director mine, Loder said, "Oh, Jesus, conditions were bad. No ventilation…. I saw it down there on the 400 and… a match wouldn't burn. You had to walk five or six hundred feet out in the drift back towards the shaft to get bit of air."[27]

According to Loder, dust was a constant problem, as were the persistent headaches that plagued him and many others. Conditions were made worse, he said, by the increase in production throughout the 1950s, when the mine was run on three shifts a day with no break between shifts. Men going down for their shift entered a workplace filled with smoke and dust from the work carried out at the end of the previous shift. No one was issued a mask, he said, and — contrary to what the inspectorate reported — fumes from the diesel tram cars were "really bad" and clogged the nasal system with black soot.[28]

Loder also remarked that the inspection system was largely useless since the company always had enough notice of an inspection visit to deal with obvious problems temporarily and put a good face on the situation:

> [The company] knew when [the inspectors] were coming. Three or four days before they came, places that there were people working, they were taken out of it, and when they were gone they were back

> in there again.... Everything would be tidied up and there'd be signs up here and signs up there.[29]

The apparent laxity towards employers was in sharp contrast to how enforcement authorities dealt with workers who violated the legislation. In 1955, two St. Lawrence miners who lit a fire to help strip hose fittings underground were convicted for a violation of the Act, marking the only instance of anyone's being charged with a violation over the entire course of the St. Lawrence disaster (Department of Mines and Resources 1956, 100).

Identifying and Responding to Silicosis

While miners continued to contend with increasing hazards that the government and the employers took no measures to address, the health effects of the working environment were becoming clearer and more pervasive during the late 1940s and early 1950s. Suspicions that health hazards in the mines were beginning to take their toll were heightened by an apparently high incidence of tuberculosis among workers and their atypical reaction to standard treatments.

Herbert Slaney, Adrian's brother, was unusual among men at St. Lawrence in that he was able to attend high school in St. John's in the late 1940s. He often visited patients from his hometown at the tuberculosis sanitarium, where there were often more than twenty St. Lawrence miners at one time. It became so common for St. Lawrence miners to be admitted to the sanitarium that people began referring to their condition as "miners' TB." Herbert Slaney said he and others were also struck by the fact that these men seemed not to respond to treatment as others did and seemed to die at a higher rate than usual among tuberculosis victims.[30]

Adrian Slaney recalled a similar scenario. When he went to visit his uncle at the sanitarium in 1950, he said, there were "all these men from St. Lawrence, and the ones who were there before had come home and died, while men from other places treated for TB were recovering." One former tuberculosis patient, he recalled, even went back to work at the mine and died two months later. As Adrian Slaney put it, it was obvious by the early 1950s that St. Lawrence miners were dying, but "we didn't know what they were dying from."[31]

The answer began to emerge in 1950 when Dr. J.J. Pepper, one of several physicians who had passed through the community over the years, examined the x-rays of an ailing miner named Issac Slaney. These x-rays had been taken by a travelling health clinic that visited isolated communities as part of the anti-tuberculosis campaign ongoing at this time. Pepper sent the x-rays to a colleague in Ottawa, who agreed with his assessment that the man's lungs showed signs of silicosis as well as tuberculosis.

Tuberculosis often created confusion about the connection between lung ailments and working conditions, as it had among miners in the U.S. and in Great Britain during the early twentieth century (Derickson 1998b, 66–89; Bryder 1985, 108–26). In fact, a definite pathological connection between tuberculosis and silicosis had been established by this time, for it had been recognized that silicosis reduces the capacity of the respiratory system to combat the effects of tuberculosis-causing germs. The term "silico-tuberculosis" had evolved to describe the resulting condition.

Believing that there were other similar cases among miners and former miners at St. Lawrence, Pepper wrote the Department of National Health and Welfare asking for help in starting a health survey among the miners. He was told that the federal department would act on such a request only if it were put to them by the provincial Department of Health (Ayward 1969, 34).

In the report on his 1950 inspection, A.V. Corlett, the mines inspector brought in from Ontario, discussed the diagnosis of Issac Slaney's condition at some length and disputed it on several grounds. Challenging a medical diagnosis appeared to lie outside Corlett's mandate as an inspector; in addition, many of his objections resulted from a failure to take into account variations in the length of exposure required to develop silicosis and the length of time between exposure and diagnosis of the disease. The exposure time required to develop silicosis varies greatly, from less than five years up to forty years, depending on the severity of the exposure and other factors. Long after dust exposure has ceased, moreover, retention of silica dust in the lungs has been known to create silicosis (Gibbs and Pintus 1978, 76–78). Because his assessment did not include such considerations, Corlett suggested that it was "highly unlikely that a miner would contract silicosis in the extremely wet mines that prevail at St. Lawrence," and he pointed out that "wet drilling is practiced at St. Lawrence." He discussed, however, conditions that prevailed in some St. Lawrence mines in 1950, not those prevalent in the 1930s and early 1940s when Issac Slaney had worked there.[32]

Questioning the procedure by which the case had been diagnosed, Corlett requested the opinion of Dr. Bennett at the sanitarium in St. John's. Bennett replied that sanitarium doctors lacked sufficient experience with silicosis to confirm or deny the diagnosis. Corlett described this response as "entirely at variance with the statements offered in St. Lawrence," which of course it was not. Corlett then contacted Dr. Riddell at the Ontario Workmen's Compensation Board (WCB). Like Bennett, Riddell replied that he was unable to confirm the diagnosis one way or the other, which Corlett again wrongly described as a rejection of Pepper's initial diagnosis.

While Corlett conceded that there was a higher than usual incidence of tuberculosis at St. Lawrence, he suggested that it was not related to mining.

Furthermore, he claimed that "the attitude that any man who has worked in a mine and who develops tuberculosis must be a silicosis victim is unfair to the mining industry." Corlett acknowledged that discussions with the mine operators and with the doctor indicated that samples taken underground revealed potentially harmful levels of dust, but dismissed this evidence on the grounds that it was "improbable that any dust in the mine picked up as a sample would yield any useful information." Nonetheless, Corlett suggested that it might be prudent to "pay attention to mine ventilation in the St. Lawrence area" because a change in conditions might require the removal of "dangerous concentrations of dust."[33]

Dr. Pepper, however, continued to pursue the matter. When Issac Slaney died in December 1952, at the age of forty-six, Pepper asked Herbert Slaney to pick up a package for him when he visited his wife in the hospital at Burin, where she had recently given birth. The package contained surgical and other equipment to which Pepper did not have access at the makeshift clinic at St. Lawrence. Pepper then convinced Rennie Slaney, the father of Adrian and Herbert and a mine captain with the St. Lawrence Corporation, to stand witness while he obtained a lung sample from Issac Slaney's corpse. Herbert Slaney was to stay outside the door to Issac Slaney's living room, where the traditional wake was going on, in order to prevent anyone from entering while Pepper performed the procedure. Pepper then sent the sample of Issac Slaney's lung tissue to an expert in the United States, who confirmed that it was silicotic.[34]

Now under increasing pressure to formulate a response to the St. Lawrence situation, officials of the Newfoundland Department of Mines, the Department of Health and Welfare, and the Newfoundland WCB met late in 1953 to discuss a strategy. A major influence on their thinking was the fact that as part of the legislative changes that accompanied confederation with Canada in 1950 the provincial government had passed Newfoundland's first compulsory, collective workers compensation legislation; this Act, like others across the country, listed silicosis as a compensable illness for those employed in mining. Apprehension over the financial implications of widespread industrial disease for the mining companies was indicated in one of the conclusions of that 1953 meeting: "the welfare of the residents of a mining community must be weighed against the possible financial liability of the mine owners should silicosis become prevalent to the point where heavy compensation is necessary."[35]

Compounding the concern about the potential financial implications of compensation claims for employers was anxiety over job losses that might result from certain options. For example, shortly after attending the 1953 meeting with WCB and Department of Mines officials, Newfoundland's Deputy Minister of Health, Leonard Miller, contacted G.C. Brink at the federal Department of Health and Welfare to express concern over a "possible" case of silicosis in St. Lawrence. As he told Brink, Miller was aware that Ontario had instituted a system of pre-employment and annual testing for respiratory ailments among miners in 1928, but he was concerned that introducing such a system at St. Lawrence might cause many workers to lose their jobs.[36] Brink simply replied that in Ontario, pre-employment and annual screening combined with adequate ventilation had been found to reduce silicosis; he suggested that all miners and former miners at St. Lawrence be given x-rays immediately.[37]

Instead of acting on this advice, the government apparently chose to continue its public relations efforts. The St. Lawrence Corporation manager told the union in 1954 that, according to information he had received from the Chief Inspector, "a man would have to work for 197 years in our mines, under our worst conditions, to accumulate sufficient silica in his lungs to exceed the 'safe' amount."[38]

However, some in St. Lawrence did not share Poynter's confidence. In March 1954, Rennie Slaney, who had witnessed the Issac Slaney autopsy, wrote to Dr. Bennett at the St. John's sanitarium regarding his brother, who was a patient there. Rennie Slaney stated that his brother had worked with dry drills at the St. Lawrence Corporation mines during the 1930s and that, even after wet drills were introduced in most St. Lawrence mines after 1941, conditions were very bad because of inadequate ventilation. He listed four St. Lawrence miners who had died after being treated at the sanitarium, nine others who were currently in the sanitarium, and several others who were never admitted to hospital but had died from undetermined "lung trouble." According to Rennie Slaney, once they had become ill, these men, like his uncle, "were cut off from any financial assistance from the company, although some had given up to 20 years of service."[39] Bennett forwarded Slaney's letter to Miller, who forwarded it to Mines Minister Fred Rowe. There is no evidence of a response.

Apart from holding meetings, downplaying fears, and soliciting advice from outside experts upon which it did not act, the Newfoundland government continued to do little to address the problem.[40] In July 1954, the Department of Health received the results of the latest tuberculosis survey, which showed that the incidence of tuberculosis in St. Lawrence was twice that of those nearby communities where most men worked in the fishery.[41] In response, government officials met again to discuss the St. Lawrence situation and agreed that the concentration of dust in the St. Lawrence Corporation mines would not likely harm "normal persons" — those not already suffering from a respiratory ailment. It was noted, however, that this conclusion was based on dust samples sent to Ottawa for examination, of which only one could be analyzed because of problems with breakage and settling during shipping. The question of employee screening arose again at this meeting but was not resolved, as officials were unsure where to draw the line for rejecting applicants or taking workers out of the mines.[42]

Dealing with possible compensation claims for silicosis also became more difficult when tuberculosis was a complicating factor. The Newfoundland WCB was uncertain of how to determine the cause of illness and the percentage of an individual's disability caused by the two ailments.[43] The matter was complicated by the fact that the 1951 Workmen's Compensation Act would only recognize cases in which disability arose after the Act came into effect, regardless of when the exposure had occurred. Because the date of disablement was considered to be the date the worker ceased working because of incapacity, anyone who had left the job before April 1, 1951, even because of an ailment covered under the Act, was not entitled to compensation. Nor were the dependents of a deceased worker who had left the job or died because of an industrial disease before April 1, 1951. As the WCB explained to the St. Lawrence Corporation manager, "The whole silicosis thing is very complicated from the legal standpoint and also because of factors like TB."[44] In the case of Issac Slaney, for example, because he had terminated his employment before the Workmen's Compensation Act came into force, the only recourse for his widow was to sue the St. Lawrence Corporation. The widow did in fact sue and settled with the company out of court for a cash payment.[45]

In the midst of this increasing awareness of industrial disease came a development with important implications for addressing this problem. In 1954 the community finally received a hospital. The facility was a gift from the American government to the people of St. Lawrence and the nearby town of Lawn who had rescued the crew of the warships that ran aground in the area in 1942. Ironically, while the union and others in the community had long been lobbying the Newfoundland government and the mining companies for help in establishing medical facilities, the hospital came from a foreign government and was the result of yet more sacrifice and work on the part of local people.

In May 1955, the Newfoundland WCB met with the Ontario WCB to discuss a number of matters: the procedure for establishing a Silicosis Referee Board in Newfoundland based on the Ontario model, the question of mines inspections and dust control in mines, a chest survey of St. Lawrence miners, and possible amendments to the relevant Newfoundland legislation.[46] Apparently little action resulted. More than a year later, the SLWPU told the Department of Mines and the Department of Health that there had been several deaths among St. Lawrence miners in the past year and that five others had been diagnosed with silicosis and tuberculosis. The union claimed the situation had become "extremely urgent" and implored the government to take immediate action to investigate the health of miners and former miners as well as conditions in the mines.[47]

The 1957 Dust Study

The government clearly did not share the union's sense of urgency. In February 1957, the Chief Inspector of Mines noted that that the first phase of a three-phase plan formulated four years earlier had now been completed: a meeting had been held among representatives of the WCB and the departments of Health and Mines on the matter of employee screening, and mine operators had submitted their comments on the issue. The American Smelting and Refining Company, which ran the lead and zinc mines at Buchans, had declined comment. The Dominion Steel and Coal Corporation, operators of the Bell Island iron ore mines, suggested that older employees be exempted from the annual examination process for fear of losing employment and suffering financial hardship and that prospective employees be required to obtain a certificate only after being hired. The Iron Ore Company of Canada, operators of mines in Labrador, suggested that mine managers be given the right to decide what a "dust exposure occupation" was. Newfluor and the St. Lawrence Corporation suggested that an annual examination was unnecessary and that a worker found to be suffering from a respiratory disease simply be taken off the job by a physician.[48]

Even the Department of Mines — which had not distinguished itself as a champion of health and safety — considered the suggestion by Newfluor and the St. Lawrence Corporation unacceptable, since workers would be taken off the job only when they became obviously ill. The Department suggested instead that annual examinations of workers already on the job should consider only tuberculosis as grounds for disqualification from continued employment but that during pre-employment screening, any respiratory disease should be grounds for disqualification.[49] This was obviously an attempt to curtail mass disqualifications among St. Lawrence miners, as it would allow those with silicosis and other ailments already on the job to remain there.

Meanwhile, many workers at the St. Lawrence Corporation would soon lose their jobs in any case, since that company entered a period of decline after the expiry of the four-year supply contract it had signed with the U.S. Defense Materials Procurement Agency in 1952. Anticipating that this would spell trouble for the St. Lawrence Corporation, Seibert had written to Premier Smallwood in 1955, describing the difficulties of competing on the international level and seeking government assistance to protect jobs at St. Lawrence. Seibert blamed his company's predicament primarily on the fact that producers in other nations, especially Mexico, were capturing a larger share of the Canadian and U.S. markets, a situation encouraged by the absence of import duties on foreign fluorspar coming in to Canada.[51]

The Newfoundland government apparently offered no practical assistance in response to Seibert's request and, unable to secure an alternate market, the St. Lawrence Corporation started laying off workers late in 1956. By the spring of 1957, its two main producers, Blue Beach and Iron Springs, had been phased out.[51] Other mines followed, and by the summer of 1957 only ten workers remained to provide basic maintenance (*Evening Telegram* June 6, 1957).

Closure of the St. Lawrence Corporation mines generated public concern about the future of the mining industry and the community, along with anger over foreign competition that could undercut domestic industries because "people in other parts of the world are satisfied to be ill-fed, ill clothed, ill-housed, and to live under conditions of economic slavery" (*Newfoundland Journal of Commerce* June 1957). Others pointed out that many of the 250 men who had lost their jobs at the St. Lawrence Corporation did not even have the option of returning to the fishery, since many had little experience in that industry and lacked boats and equipment (*Evening Telegram* June 8, 1957).

Closure of the St. Lawrence Corporation mines also meant they escaped detailed examination when the provincial government finally took action to determine the extent of the dust hazard. Having rejected a request from Pepper seven years earlier on the grounds that it would act only at the request of the Newfoundland Department of Health, the national Department of Health and Welfare now agreed to assist the provincial department (Aylward 1969, 34). It sent an industrial hygienist from its Occupational Health and Safety Division to conduct dust surveys at St. Lawrence.

J.P. Windish arrived at St. Lawrence just two weeks after the closure of the last operating St. Lawrence Corporation mine. Unlike the earlier samples taken by the inspectorate, those Windish collected at Newfluor were analyzed within twenty-four hours of being collected. The analysis used the standard formula under which the amount of silica dust is expressed as millions of particles per cubic foot of air, or MPPCF. For different percentages of free silica, there is a different threshold limit value (TLV), defined as "that concentration of a material to which, it is believed, a workman may be repeatedly exposed day after day without suffering demonstrable physiological damage." For the percentage of free silica in the dust samples taken at Newfluor, it was determined that the TLV was 20 MPPCF (Sanderson and Windish 1958, 6).

Several readings taken during drilling operations on the 550-foot level of the Director mine, where no mechanical ventilation had been provided, were in excess of the limit. Windish noted that while these readings were not highly excessive, the dust was especially harmful because the drill was often directly above the driller's face. He also pointed out that the high readings on the 550-foot level were in an extremely wet area, indicating that contrary

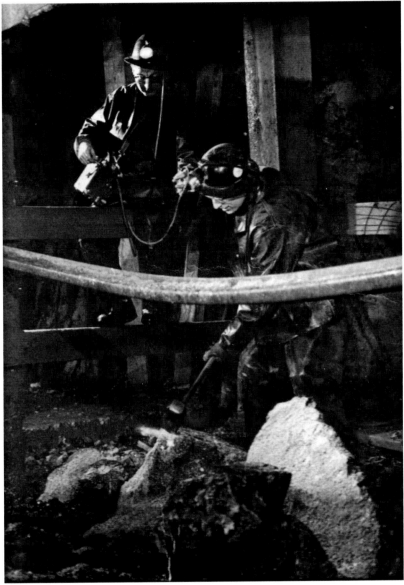

J.P. Windish taking an air sample in Director mine, c. 1957.

to widespread belief, "the mere presence of plenty of water in an area is not sufficient to suppress dust." Readings up to thirty-five times the TLV were recorded during drilling on the 400-foot level, where stopes also had no ventilation (Sanderson and Windish 1958, 9–11). Windish noted that while at the time the mining industry commonly used drills that would not run without a supply of water, many of those used in the Director mine could

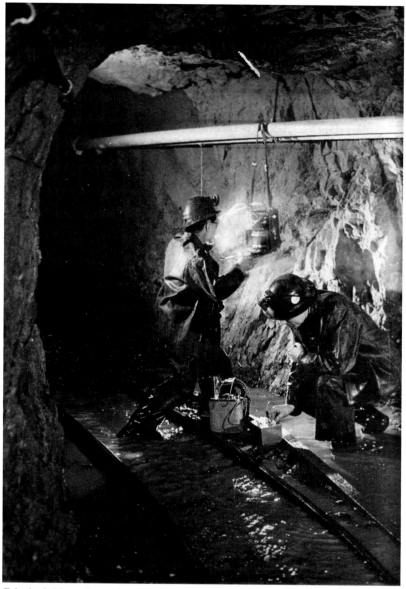

Federal technicians using smoke method to determine airflow in Director mine, c. 1957. Note the stream of water, soon found to be contaminated with radon.

be run without water (Sanderson and Windish 1958, 2–3). Readings many times the SWL (safe working level) were also generated by operations like constructing ore chutes from one level to another and blasting down ore in the stopes (Sanderson and Windish 1958, 9–11).

Nor was the dust hazard confined to underground operations. Some of the highest readings were recorded in surface operations. In the building where the ore was crushed before being conveyed to a Heavy Media Separation plant for further refining, dust that accumulated on the crusher motors and other equipment was blown off using compressed air, creating levels up to 1,200 times the TLV. Windish noted that the solution to this problem was a simple one that had been adopted at most similar operations in Canada: enclosing the equipment motors so that they did not require daily cleaning and installing ventilation equipment to remove the dust (Sanderson and Windish 1958, 15–17).

Windish's general conclusion was that there was a "serious dust hazard" associated with nearly every aspect of the underground and surface operations at Newfluor. Furthermore, he noted, the high readings at Newfluor were based on a relatively high TLV of 20 MPPCF; many Canadian and American operations had adopted 5 MPPCF as their target level in an attempt to reduce the silicosis risk (Sanderson and Windish 1958, 18–19). Regarding the possible health effects of these conditions, Windish observed: "The ultimate criterion against which the hazard of the working environment must be assessed will of course be the health of the miners after, say, 20 years of exposure to mining conditions" (Sanderson and Windish 1958, 18).

Confirming what many at St. Lawrence had been saying for years, the 1957 dust survey provided further evidence of a link between working conditions and ailments such as like silicosis and silico-tuberculosis. It also highlighted the government's negligence in failing to enforce the legislation and Newfluor's disregard for their workers' health. The evidence offers little reason to believe that dust levels at the operations of the St. Lawrence Corporation would have been better. As bad as matters were with respect to dust and dust-induced diseases, however, events would soon show that the situation was even more horrendous than anyone had imagined.

Notes

1. History of Operations, 1966, AA.
2. Warren S. Smith, Fluorspar at St. Lawrence, Newfoundland, 1957 File 1 L/4/16, DME.
3. Warren S. Smith, Fluorspar at St. Lawrence, Newfoundland, 1957 File 1 L/4/16, DME.
4. Howard Farrell, Report of the Mining Properties of St. Lawrence Corporation, 1967, File 1L/14, DME.
5. Walter Seibert to J.R. Smallwood, 7 November 1949, Coll 075 (Smallwood Collection), File 3.20.087, CNSA.
6. Howard Farrell, Report of the Mining Properties of St. Lawrence Corporation, 1967, File 1L/14, DME, 15–40.
7. Howard Farrell, Report of the Mining Properties of St. Lawrence Corporation, 1967, File 1L/14, DME, 15–40, 48–51.

8. Howard Farrell, Report of the Mining Properties of St. Lawrence Corporation, 1967, File 1L/14, DME, 15–40.
9. Interview with Richard Loder, 15 October 2000.
10. Interview with James Cusick, St. Lawrence, 13 October 1968. Coll 84-224, Tapes C7253-7254, MUNFLA.
11. Interview with James Cusick, MUNFLA.
12. Interview with James Cusick, MUNFLA.
13. Interview with James Cusick, MUNFLA.
14. AFL Research Staff to James Cusick, SLWPU, 12 May 1952, MM.
15. Report of the Conciliation Board in the matter of a dispute between St. Lawrence Federal Labour Union No. 24530 and the St. Lawrence Corporation of Newfoundland, Limited, 24 October 1953, MM.
16. Aloysius Turpin, SLWPU, to George Meany, President, American Federation of Labor, Washington, 12 May 1955, and Russell Harvey, Regional Director, AFL, Toronto, to Aloysius Turpin, SLWPU, 19 May 1955, MM.
17. Minutes of meeting, SLWPU, 26 March 1956, MM.
18. Inspection of Newfoundland mines for safety of workmen and operating features, submitted by A.V. Corlett, Mining Engineer, Kingston, Ontario, to Claude K. Howse, Government Geologist, Department of Natural Resources, St. John's, Newfoundland, 30 November 1949, DME.
19. A.V. Corlett, Inspection of Newfoundland mines for the safety of workmen and operating features, 1950, DME.
20. A.V. Corlett, Inspection of Newfoundland mines for the safety of workmen and operating features, 1951, DME.
20. F. Gover, Chief Inspector of Mines, to F.W. Rowe, Minister of Mines and Resources, 8 February 1953, File NFLD/0083, DME.
22. Interview with Jerome Spearns, 28 November 1998.
23. Interview with Jerome Spearns, 28 November 1998.
24. Interview with Adrian Slaney, 7 February 2000.
25. Interview with Adrian Slaney, 7 February 2000.
26. Interview with Adrian Slaney, 7 February 2000.
27. Interview with Richard Loder, 15 October 2000.
28. Interview with Richard Loder, 15 October 2000.
29. Interview with Richard Loder 15 October 2000.
30. Interview with Herbert Slaney, 13 October 2000.
31. Interview with Adrian Slaney, 7 February 2000.
32. A.V. Corlett, Inspection of Newfoundland mines for the safety of workmen and operating features, 1950, DME.
33. A.V. Corlett, Inspection of Newfoundland mines for the safety of workmen and operating features, 1950, DME.
34. Interview with Herbert Slaney, 13 October 2000.
35. Proceedings of meeting on the subject of detection and handling of silicosis held in the office of the Chief Inspector of Mines, 30 October 1953, GN 78/1/B, 51, PANL.
36. Miller to G.C. Brink, Department of Health and Welfare, Ottawa, 10 November 1953, GN 78/1/B, 51, PANL.
37. Brink to Miller, 19 November 1953, GN 78/1/B, 51, PANL.

38. Donald Poynter, St. Lawrence Corporation of Newfoundland, to Gregory Giovaninni, Acting President, SLWPU, 25 October 1954, MM.
39. Rennie Slaney, St. Lawrence, to Dr. R.B. Bennett, Superintendent of St. John's Sanitarium, 25 March 1954, GN 78/1/B, 51, PANL.
40. C.R. Ross, Industrial Hygiene Engineer, Department of Health and Welfare, Ottawa, to Miller, 23 June 1954, GN 78/1/B, 51, PANL.
41. BCG Testing and Vaccination, July 1954, GN 78/1/B, 51, PANL.
42. Meeting of Committee on Silicosis, 19 August 1954, GN 78/1/B, 51, PANL.
43. WCB of Ontario, to Irving Fogwill, Chairman of WCB of Newfoundland, 31 August 1954, GN 78/1/B, 51, PANL.
44. Irving Fogwill, WCB, to Donald Poynter, St. Lawrence Corporation, 13 November 1954, GN 78/1/B, 51, PANL.
45. Case Files, Royal Commission on St. Lawrence, GN 6, 1, PANL.
46. Irving Fogwill, Agenda for Toronto meeting proposed for 2 May 1955, 5 April 1955, GN 78/1/B, 51, PANL.
47. P.J. Lewis to W.J. Keough, Deputy Minister of Mines, and to Miller, 30 August 1956, GN 78/1/B, 51, PANL.
48. B. Lukins, Chief Inspector of Mines, to Leonard Miller, Newfoundland Department of Health, and to Irving Fogwill, Workers' Compensation Board, 27 February 1957, GN 78/1/B, 51, File 290/G/07, PANL.
49. Lukins to Miller and to Fogwill, 27 February 1957, GN 78/1/B, 51, File 290/G/07, PANL.
50. Walter Seibert, St. Lawrence Corporation, to Smallwood, 27 December 1955, Coll 075, File 3.20.087, CNSA.
51. Howard Farrell, Report of the Mining Properties of St. Lawrence Corporation, 1967, File 1L/14, DME, 24–47.

Chapter Four

MORE DEADLY PERILS
Radiation and Cancer

Revelations of the Tariff Hearing

The animosity the union president had come to harbour for the St. Lawrence Corporation is indicated by his reaction to a January 1958 announcement that the Canadian Tariff Board would conduct an inquiry into the issue of imposing a tariff on fluorspar entering Canada (Canada Department of Finance 1958, 7). Turpin noted that while the union was pleased that the outcome might help his members get their jobs back, it was ambivalent about the prospect of assisting Seibert and the company:

> We the people are fed up with the St. Lawrence Corporation of Newfoundland Limited, and at times feel you are only fighting a battle for Seibert, who's not after all worth fighting for.... His old shoestring and penny-pinching are still with us, and the rank and file, my union men see no future under [that management]. We didn't see it in 1941, and no better today, only worse.... conditions were of the worst at all times, and you know all his faithful friends or employees got silicosis.[1]

Government representatives also criticized Seibert for doing nothing but wait for the Tariff Board's ruling while the government and the union attempted to find a solution to the crisis. Deputy Minister of Mines Fred Gover suggested that many of the St. Lawrence Corporation's difficulties resulted from running its operation in a badly planned manner with substandard equipment.[2] Curiously, Gover had levelled no such criticisms while serving as Chief Inspector of Mines several years previous.

While the union was naturally concerned about the outcome, Turpin declined to participate in or even make a written submission to the tariff hearing that was held in Ottawa in May 1957, claiming that he and other members of the union executive were not qualified to address such a complex issue.[3] At the hearing, the St. Lawrence Corporation requested a tariff of $10 per ton on fluorspar imported into Canada. For obvious reasons, fluorspar consumers, a group that included Algoma Steel, Atlas Steels, the Steel Company of Canada (Stelco) of Ontario, and Dosco of Nova Scotia, opposed any tariff. Alcan, because it produced fluorspar only for its own use, also opposed a tariff on the grounds that it might increase production costs should Alcan ever have to import foreign fluorspar and might invoke retaliatory tariffs from countries where it sold its aluminum products. Based on these arguments and on the fact that a reasonable level of tariff could not counteract the much lower cost of producing fluorspar in Mexico, the Board denied the request for a tariff (Canada, Department of Finance 1958, 32–34).

The hearings also provided some significant revelations about the activities of the St. Lawrence Corporation, both local and international. Seibert stated that the St. Lawrence Corporation had made a profit every year from 1936 to 1956, and that the years 1954 to 1956 were especially prosperous, once again casting doubt on the company's repeated claims that it was in no position to improve wages or working conditions (Canada, Department of Finance 1958, Appendix C). Furthermore, testimony from consumers indicated that at the same time the St. Lawrence Corporation had been bemoaning the effect of cheap fluorspar from Mexico on its St. Lawrence operation, it had in fact been attempting to market Mexican fluorspar to Canadian consumers. The St. Lawrence Corporation, it turned out, was a major investor in a Mexican fluorspar mining company known as Compania Minera Julieta, which had been operating a mine in northern Mexico for several years, and Seibert had been seeking markets among Canadian consumers for fluorspar from that mine. Stelco, for example, stated that the St. Lawrence Corporation had offered to supply it with "Mexican fluorspar" in 1955, 1956, and 1957. Dosco stated that the St. Lawrence Corporation had quoted it a price on Mexican flourspar in 1955, saying it could be supplied "through their Mexican connections." Algoma testified that in 1954, 1955, and 1956, offers of "Mexican fluorspar" were made "from St. Lawrence Corporation's associated producer in Mexico" (Canada, Department of Finance 1958, 24–25).

The St. Lawrence Corporation's involvement with the Mexican producer raises the question of why Seibert requested the tariff in the first place. What could he hope to gain by having a tariff imposed on that fluorspar? One possible explanation is that the geology of the Mexican mine, combined with the price of labour there, made exporting fluorspar profitable even with a tariff, as was pointed out during the hearing. The Tariff Board suggested that Seibert might have been after a tariff sufficient to allow for a small profit within the Canadian market, which would help subsidize re-entry into the more profitable U.S. acid-grade market. The Tariff Board conceded, however, that the St. Lawrence Corporation's finances were so convoluted as to make any informed judgment on its motives impossible.

Revelations about Seibert's activities in the Mexican fluorspar industry fuelled the animosity toward him and the St. Lawrence Corporation. Turpin was outraged that St. Lawrence men were "walking about dying of silicosis" while Seibert was investing in the Mexican fluorspar industry to put them out of work.[4] Seibert attempted to placate Turpin by assuring him that his Mexican dealings had nothing to do with the shutdown in St. Lawrence and that closing the St. Lawrence mines was "tearing my heart out as I know many of our faithful employees who have been with us for many years are going to suffer financially and otherwise."[5]

The Newfoundland government, meanwhile, reacted to the ruling by cobbling together a plan to get the St. Lawrence Corporation mines running again, at least on a limited and temporary basis, by guaranteeing a line of credit for $200,000 to reactivate the most promising mines on a small scale.[6] Collateral would be the ore itself, with the money advanced in installments based on the market value of ore as it was produced.[7] This response was no doubt related to the fact that the province was in the throes of a recession, with unemployment moving towards its highest level since the 1930s.

Turpin greeted the news that the company would restart mining with a mixture of relief and skepticism: he was glad some men would return to work, but hoped that the Department of Mines would take the opportunity to enforce health and safety laws "in order that our miners may live longer."[8]

Cancer and Conflict, 1958–1962

By the time the results of the 1957 dust study were made public in May 1958, concern was shifting to another and possibly more horrendous problem: an apparently high rate of lung cancer among miners. In January 1958, for instance, Turpin indicated local awareness of this matter when he noted to the chair of a cancer convention being held in St. John's that "a large number of our miners died with Cancer and Silicosis."[9] By June of that year, provincial health authorities were also becoming concerned with this issue. Deputy Minister of Health Leonard Miller contacted federal health authorities and Alcan's Chief Industrial Medical Officer, Frank Brent, regarding the "altogether disproportionate number of deaths from carcinoma of the lung" among St. Lawrence miners and requested any information or advice they might offer.[10] Miller noted that of fourteen male deaths from carcinoma of the lung in Newfoundland in 1956, three were St. Lawrence miners and two of these had been in their early forties.[11]

While federal authorities agreed that this appeared an abnormally high rate, they could point to no known connection between cancer and the mining of fluorspar.[12] Brent said that he had noticed what seemed to him a high cancer rate among miners during a visit to St. Lawrence in 1957, but could offer no explanation for it. However, he was careful to point out that though some of the men so far believed to have died from cancer had worked for Newfluor, all of them had worked for the St. Lawrence Corporation at some point.[13] Corporate interests were already maneuvering to reduce their culpability in this latest chapter of the unfolding disaster.

To help gather more information on the matter, the provincial government once again turned to the Occupational Health Division of the federal Department of Health and Welfare. Based on information gathered on several visits during 1958 and 1959, Industrial Hygienist Dr. A.J. deVilliers proposed a detailed study on occupational hazards at the mines.[14] Miller advised federal authorities to proceed with this study as soon as possible since the union, spurred by the mounting death toll had been strongly lobbying him and other provincial officials.[15] In November 1959, Turpin told Newfoundland Labour Minster Charles Ballam that "The bell still tolls, two more miners [just] died of cancer of the lung."[16]

A study into a possible workplace source of cancer was begun in November 1959 under the direction of J.P. Windish, who had conducted the 1957 dust survey. While pleased that officials were finally taking some action, the union noted that in the twenty years since workers had started asking for such help, "half the membership" had died or were ill, many of these had never been compensated, and widows and children were left to survive by whatever means they could, usually welfare.[17]

Windish focused on radiation as the likely cancer-causing agent, and tests conducted from November 1959 to January 1960 revealed concentrations of the radioactive gas radon-222 "much in excess of the currently accepted maximum permissible concentration in all levels of the Director mine" (Windish 1960, 1–2). The accessible portions of the St. Lawrence Corporation mines were also found to contain dangerously high levels of radiation.[18] The solid "radon daughters" created by the decay of radon-222 became attached to dust or condensation in the air and were deposited on the lungs when inhaled. Depending on the concentration and duration of exposure, these radon daughters often led to the development of cancer, particularly of the lungs (Windish 1960, 12–13).

Windish's observations also revealed that inadequate ventilation contributed to the hazard. At Director mine, concentrations varied from below SWL in some places up to 193 times the SWL in others because of different levels of ventilation. For instance, Windish noted that in one drift on the 550-foot level where a very high reading was obtained, there was no ventilation of any kind and "there was not enough oxygen present to support combustion" (Windish 1960, 13). An experiment he conducted showed a dramatic increase in radon concentrations as the airflow from a temporary ventilating system was gradually reduced. The lowest group of readings, on the other hand, was from the 250-foot level where mechanical ventilation had been installed to deal with exhaust from diesel locomotives. The rest of the mine was either unventilated or ventilated by limited natural draft, and Windish recommended that mechanical ventilation be installed in all underground working areas of all mines (Windish 1960, 5).

As for the source of the radon gas, there was no indication of exposed uranium in the mine, and tests did not indicate any radioactivity in the fluorspar itself. Windish therefore concluded that the radon originated outside and was carried into the mine through the groundwater — the same water miners had been drinking for years (Windish 1960, 8). (It was later confirmed that areas adjacent to the mine sites held low-grade uranium deposits.)

While radioactivity was uncommon in non-uranium mines, it was not unheard of. For example, a 1953 study revealed dangerously high levels of radon in several metal, clay, and coal mines in Colorado, and a 1954 study reported similar findings in several non-uranium mines in New York State (Jacoe 1953; Harris 1954, 54–60). Windish himself cited such cases as evidence that the existence of radon gas in the Director mine was not an "extraordinary or unique occurrence" (Windish 1960, 23). What distinguished St. Lawrence was that the concentration of radon there was considerably higher than that reported in other non-uranium mines up to that time, and six times higher than the highest reading obtained in any non-uranium mine in the United States (Windish 1960, 23).

Provincial authorities and the employers — but not the union or the workers — were informed of the findings in December 1959. At this point, Brent became more concerned with controlling the flow of information. For example, he insisted that Newfoundland Health Minister James McGrath make no public statements without first informing the company. He also sought confirmation from McGrath that the two had agreed that there existed no "proof positive" of a link between cancer and working conditions at St. Lawrence.[19]

The Newfoundland government also faced the challenge of how to meet another of Windish's recommendations: that a system be established to monitor the radiation hazard. This matter is best understood in the broader context of how the issue had evolved in Canada up to that point. Since the establishment of the first uranium mines in the early 1930s, successive Canadian governments had sought to keep the nuclear industry under exclusive federal control, partly through the creation of crown corporations such as Eldorado Nuclear in 1944 and Atomic Energy Canada Limited (AECL) in 1952, and the 1946 establishment of the Atomic Energy Control Board (AECB), a regulatory body with sweeping powers over the nuclear industry, including uranium mining. In the early 1950s, with the uranium mining industry expanding, some provinces — notably Ontario — complained that efforts to develop the industry were being hampered by the fact that while in other types of mines health and safety was a provincial matter, the federal government controlled this and all other aspects of the uranium mining industry. In 1955, federal and provincial authorities established an arrangement under which health and safety in uranium mines came under provincial jurisdiction while national and international authorities set standards in such areas as safe working levels.

While this may have helped clarify the jurisdictional matter, it also handed jurisdiction for a serious and complex health hazard over to provincial authorities often ill-prepared or reluctant to deal with the issue adequately (Robinson 1982, 7). That the arrangement did little to protect workers' health in Ontario, the province that pushed hardest for it, eventually became apparent when over 200 miners died from lung cancer caused by exposure to radon gas in Ontario uranium mines. The arrangement also left provinces like Newfoundland, which had never dealt with such a matter before, at a loss as to how to proceed. Miller himself conceded that the province lacked the means and the knowledge to meet Windish's recommendation.

As for the union, its reaction to the revelations about radiation was clearly shaped by its experience with past handling of occupational health issues. Shortly after workers learned of the problem in March 1960, Mines Minister W.J. Keough noted that they were doubtful the ventilation and monitoring issues would be quickly and adequately addressed — a concern based on "alleged tardiness" on the part of the employers in the past "to take steps to ensure the welfare of mineworkers at St. Lawrence." Keough urged McGrath to help clarify the matter of federal versus provincial jurisdiction and remarked, tellingly, that he hoped that both would not be involved since "one enforcing authority is enough for mine operators to have to contend with" — an attitude unlikely to produce the most desirable results with respect to health and safety.[20]

Revelations about radiation in the mines also drew unprecedented media and public attention to the St. Lawrence situation and sparked a war of words in the press. St. John's newspapers were soon reporting on the fact that radon in some parts of the Director mine was nearly 200 times the permissible level and that an average of three miners had died of cancer each year since 1948 (*Daily News* March 2, 1960, 3, 16; *Evening Telegram* March 2, 1960, 2). The national media also picked up on the story, with the *Financial Post* running a piece on cancer among St. Lawrence miners, though it shied away from drawing a definitive link to radiation in the mines (McArthur March 12, 1960).

Other parties soon weighed in. In addition to being Poynter's brother-in-law, Theo Etchegary was a supervisor with the St. Lawrence Corporation and the town mayor. It is unclear in which capacity he was speaking when he claimed that, "The men knew all along this condition existed and considered it an ordinary hazard of mining." The fact that the mayor was a member of company management meant the absence of a potential advocate who might have spoken on the part of the workers. Etchegary was supported in his view by St. Lawrence Corporation Mine Captain Murdock Judson, who claimed that the men knew that such hazards were "all part of the game" (*Evening Telegram* March 3, 1960). Such statements beg the question of how workers could have known about and accepted radiation as an inherent health risk since it had only been discovered at St. Lawrence three months earlier and it had never been known to exist in a fluorspar mine up to that time.

The union was clearly in no mood for more talk and delays. A week after learning of the hazards, all but one of the underground workers supported a motion to walk off the job and stay off until adequate ventilation was installed. Over half of the nearly 200 underground workers at both companies walked out. Of these, 84 were from Newfluor's total workforce of 143 and 22 from the St. Lawrence Corporation's workforce of 46.[21] Turpin stated that he was especially proud of the men for making this move, since the union had no strike fund (*Evening Telegram* March 11, 1960, 3; *Daily News* March 11, 1960, 3). The union vowed that underground workers would stay off the job until adequate ventilation was installed and a monitoring system established, but agreed to Newfluor's request to allow some men to enter Director mine on a rotating basis to help prepare for installing the ventilation equipment. The St. Lawrence Corporation, meanwhile, was reportedly getting its blower fans "out of storage" and planning to install them at its operating mines.[22]

About a week into the dispute, Newfluor management attempted to downplay the danger, stating that the situation was not as bad as initially described and that the survey had shown radiation levels "slightly above" the limit on one level, a direct contradiction of the information contained in the Windish report (*Evening Telegram* March 18, 1960, 46). Newfluor manager Ron Wiseman also claimed that most of the fear associated with the situation had been caused by a "distortion of the facts by the press" (*Daily News* March 18, 1960, 2). Theo Etchegary insisted that there was still no conclusive proof that radiation in the mines was linked to cancer deaths among the workers. Again, it was unclear whether he was speaking as mayor or as St. Lawrence Corporation supervisor. The union was not swayed or reassured by such talk, and the men continued to insist that they simply would not return until their demands were met (*Evening Telegram* March 24, 1960, 3).

Poynter also claimed that the situation had been exaggerated. Responding to a letter from the Unemployment Insurance Commission regarding the striking workers, Poynter suggested that the announcement about radiation levels had created unnecessary panic. "Over the years," he stated, "we have had the rare case of silicosis blamed on conditions here, and as a result we have, in conjunction with the Inspection Division of the Mines Department in St. John's and the Federal Health boys in Ottawa, kept a better than average watch on dust conditions, and we have invariably been given a clean bill of health." He acknowledged that the radiation survey had found some "odd spots" in some St. Lawrence Corporation mines, but claimed that the results were erratic and inconsistent. The one spot where radiation was found in an operating St. Lawrence Corporation mine, he stated, was blocked off "and of no importance." Poynter also remarked, cryptically, that in other mines where radiation had been found, "Everyone has level-headedly tackled the problem as we were and there has been no problem."

Poynter continued to deny a connection between working conditions and disease, stating that, "We had a tendency to believe, and still believe, that the troubles were based on an abnormal rate of T.B." He added, dismissively, that once they got their fans out of storage there would be sufficient ventilation to "blow all those nasty little radiation bugs clear out to sea [and] we hope then that one of the Ottawa boys will come in, read his magic instruments, and make the electrifying announcement that the place is now safe, then everybody will return to work."[23]

By late March, both companies were exerting pressure on the government to help end the walkout. Claiming that orders for 20,000 tons of fluorspar had to be filled, Poynter demanded to know how much ventilation his company was required to install and who would then assure the men that it was safe to return to work.[24] Similarly, Newfluor Manager Wiseman informed the Department of Mines that temporary fans had been installed on the 400-foot level in response to the "alleged" radiation hazard and that his company believed that no radiation hazard now existed in areas where men would be asked to work. Like Poynter, Wiseman wanted the safety of the workplace confirmed "so that we can contact [the union] and avoid any further unnecessary delays."[25]

Shortly after management made this request, Windish contacted the union with the results of a radiation survey conducted at the St. Lawrence Corporation and the Newfluor mines. Tests had produced one excessive figure at Director, which Windish claimed was an anomaly in an unused area and therefore not considered significant (*Evening Telegram* April 1, 1960, 3). However, Windish's assessment included an important caveat: because of "time limitations," he had taken samples only in those places mine officials had told him men would be asked to work. One area where samples were not taken was the 550-level at Director, where Windish was told no men would be working when production resumed.[26] While Windish did not explain the time limitations, presumably they reflected the desire to get back into production as soon as possible.

The first of the underground workers began returning to their jobs on April 5, when the walkout officially ended.[27] However, not all who had walked out returned: about thirty Newfluor men refused to go back. Wiseman charged that these men were simply "scared" for no reason. He may have been trying to goad the men into returning, since Newfluor was apparently having trouble finding experienced miners in order to meet its annual production target. About a hundred experienced workers had lost their jobs at the St. Lawrence Corporation, but the union claimed that Newfluor wanted no responsibility for them should they have been exposed to radiation with their former employer (*Evening Telegram* April 7, 1960). Apparently, the St. Lawrence Corporation did not encounter the same difficulty as Newfluor in getting its men back, and according to Poynter, "distorted stories" in the press about workers refusing to return to their jobs did not apply to his company.[28]

Following the walkout, work resumed on a limited basis at some of the St. Lawrence Corporation's smaller mines, such as Hare's Ears, Haypook, and Red Head. Ore produced from these mines was shipped via the Wilmington plant to American consumers.[29] Anticipating an increase in demand for 1961 and seeking to make up for time lost during the walkout, Newfluor moved quickly to put the Director mine back into full production. By July 1960, it was once again running on three shifts a day and employed about two hundred men (*Evening Telegram* April 11, 1960, 3).

The resumption of mining coincided roughly with the implementation of new provisions for medical screening of applicants and workers, which government and industry officials had been discussing since 1953. The provisions required that all applicants for employment in a dust-exposure occupation be declared by a Medical Examiner to be "free from active disease of the respiratory organs," to have no known history of active tuberculosis, and to be otherwise fit for employment in such an occupation. Once an initial certificate was obtained, annual examinations were to be required to keep it in good standing. For annual renewal, however, the holder would simply have to be free of tuberculosis of the respiratory organs. The Medical Examiner could therefore issue an annual renewal even if an employee had contracted silicosis or some other respiratory disease since the initial certificate was issued, provided the employee was free from tuberculosis. In addition, the requirements did not apply to anyone who had been "continuously employed in a dust exposure operation since the date of coming into force of this regulation" — in other words, they did not apply to current employees (*Newfoundland* September 29, 1959). Clearly, the provisions were concerned as much with keeping as many St. Lawrence miners as possible on the job as they were with addressing the health concern.

The end of the walkout did not settle the matter of radiation control and monitoring. Just a month after the men returned to work, for example, the union complained to the Chief Inspector of Mines that, contrary to Newfluor's earlier assurances, men were in fact working on the unventilated 550-foot level and that ventilation was still inadequate in many parts of the mine.[30] The union's claims were soon validated by follow-up tests conducted by Windish, which confirmed the inadequacy of ventilation at both Director and the St. Lawrence Corporation mines, especially on the 550-foot level at Director.[31]

Sources of grievance continued to mount. In the summer of 1960, a worker was killed at the Director mine. Turpin continued to complain to the government about deplorable sanitary conditions and drinking water at the St. Lawrence Corporation mines.[32] Complaints over radiation monitoring persisted. The federal government's Occupational Health and Safety Division had agreed to assist the provincial government until someone could be trained within Newfoundland to carry out the required tests.[33] Meanwhile, radiation checks were conducted by an engineering student from Memorial University, so once the student returned to school in August 1960, even those readings stopped. The union complained that the only thing workers knew for certain about radiation levels was that in many places they were higher than permitted.[34]

In October 1960, another worker was killed in a fall at Director (Newfoundland Department of Mines and Resources 1961, 78). The inspector's report attributed the accident to "an unsafe act performed by the deceased" (Newfoundland Department of Mines and Resources 1961, 78), but the union blamed it on inadequate supervision.[35] Just a few days after this incident, another event triggered yet another walkout. When a Newfluor worker was barred from the workplace for refusing to acknowledge a routine disciplinary note, his fellow underground workers vowed to stay off the job until he was permitted back without signing the note. The company argued that the dispute should be taken up through the grievance procedure embodied in the collective agreement, but the men stayed off the job. Furthermore, the oncoming shift soon joined them and the entire group went home. No one showed up for the next shift. A total of 185 surface and underground workers were now off the job.[36]

It soon became apparent that the issue that triggered the walkout was not the actual motivation. Rather, the union was taking the opportunity to demand that two men be assigned to "slushing" (gathering broken ore from a stope with a cable-operated scoop), as had been the practice up until recently. The union claimed that the presence of a second person was a safety issue, as he generally acted as a "spotter," watching out for loose rock and other dangers in the working area (*Daily News* October 25, 1960). Management countered that it was within its rights to change mining methods and that this and the union's "many other grievances" should have been pursued through the grievance procedure.[37] The dispute was ultimately settled through arbitration and the men returned to work after two weeks off the job, with two workers on the slushers.[38]

While workers at Newfluor were apparently able to use the company's need for labour to bolster their bargaining power, St. Lawrence Corporation workers were in a different position. There, the industry and the employment situation continued to be precarious, which no doubt contributed to the union's willingness simply to hold the line during re-negotiation of the collective agreement in 1960, an outcome it described as the best possible "under present conditions."[39] The St. Lawrence Corporation continued to struggle through 1960, at the end of which it employed only forty workers.[40] The company was dealt another blow in June 1961, when Seibert died suddenly. Shortly thereafter, its operations were reduced to just one small mine, and by the end of 1961, the St. Lawrence Corporation had effectively ceased operating.[41]

The decline and shutdown of the St. Lawrence Corporation mines meant that its operations were never subjected to a new regulation that came into effect in 1961. Mine operators and managers were required to test air in working portions of mines at the request of the chief inspector and report results to the chief inspector (Newfoundland March 29, 1960). Under this new regulation, Newfluor was to begin conducting tests in April 1961 and report any radiation readings in excess of the SWL.[42] Tests were to be performed every week in areas where the previous reading had been 0.6 times the SWL or higher, every month where it had been between 0.6 and 0.3, every three months where it had been less than 0.3, and initially every week in new working places. Tests were also to be conducted by the Department of Mines "when occasion permits."

This system was problematic in a number of ways. First, the government had essentially handed responsibility for monitoring the hazard over to the company. Second, identifying and addressing a dangerous build-up of radiation was of little benefit to those already exposed. Third, the reported readings were in fact the average of a number of readings taken in a particular area over a period of time. It was thus possible to have readings both well in excess of and well below the SWL for the same area and produce an average that was below the SWL. Thus a miner working in an unventilated stope might be exposed to radiation in excess of the SWL while another working nearby might be exposed to little or no radiation, but the reported reading would be the same for both areas.

For 1961, Newfluor gathered about 280 average readings; the Department of Mines, 130. Of these, fourteen were in excess of the SWL. It was reported that in all these cases the contributing condition was identified and corrected. Some common causes given for high levels were malfunctioning fans, wrongly routed airflow, and damaged vent tubing.[43] At the end of 1961, the union was notified by the Department of Mines that it was satisfied that Newfluor was doing a good job of monitoring and controlling the radiation hazard.[44]

Despite such assurances, it appears that distrust over radiation monitoring continued to affect relations between Newfluor and its workers. According to one man who worked underground at Director during this time, it was widely believed that the company monitor could "rig" the system so the reported level would be lower than the actual one. "I didn't believe the readings that the company would take," this man recalled; "no one trusted it."[45] The company recognized that this mistrust was "affecting the efficiency of the mining operations" and sought the government's help to "counteract the unwarranted bad publicity arising out of this subject."[46] A week later, the Department complied: the Minister stated publicly that the mines at St. Lawrence were now safe and the radiation problem well under control (*Daily News* May 8, 1962, 4). Shortly thereafter, Health Minister McGrath sent the same assurances to the union's lawyer.[47]

However, labour relations continued to be strained, as was evident in another wildcat strike in 1962, again over a disciplinary matter. This time a worker nearly came to blows with a shift boss in a dispute over a minor matter.[48] At an emergency meeting, 170 union members voted unanimously to walk off the job and stay off until the shift boss was dismissed.[49] The men stayed off for seven days, returning when it was agreed to gather more evidence about the incident.[50]

Affiliation with the CNTU

In this context of escalating complaints and unrest, in 1962 the SLWPU once again sought to affiliate with an outside organization. The reasons for this might be inferred from several developments in the years since the union had broken its affiliation with the NFL/AFL in 1956. Turpin himself had conceded in 1957 that neither he nor anyone else on the union executive was competent to make a submission to the Tariff Board hearings. During the several work stoppages of the early 1960s, workers had no strike fund or outside assistance. In 1959, the union had hired a Montreal research firm to provide information on wages paid to Alcan workers at Arvida — which turned out to be an average of $1.95 per hour plus a cost-of-living bonus, compared to an average wage of just $1.55 per hour at Newfluor.[51] In 1960, Turpin had contacted the International Union of Mine, Mill and Smelter Workers seeking information on radiation hazards in mines, to which Mine-Mill responded with a report on radiation hazards at the Elliot Lake uranium mines.[52] Such incidents indicate the drawbacks in remaining independent, drawbacks that the union was beginning to see.

The higher wages paid at the Arvida plant, moreover, raised interest in the organization representing Arvida workers, the Quebec-based Confederation of National Trade Unions (CNTU). In October 1962, SLWPU workers voted overwhelmingly to request affiliation with the CNTU.[53] The CNTU replied favourably, promising to assist the SLWPU in every way possible and noting that it was "deeply impressed by the militant efforts of your local to improve the deplorable conditions of work and health hazards to which the workers of Newfoundland Fluorspar Limited are subjected."[54] When the union's new status was officially certified in January 1963, the SLWPU became the first union outside Quebec to affiliate with the CNTU.

The CNTU, one of the country's oldest labour organizations, had gone through a number of transformations over the years. According to one account, it was formed in 1921 as a "fearful response" by the Catholic Church to the increasing influence and the radicalism of international unions in Canada, and was originally sectarian and conservative in character (Black Rose Books Editorial Collective 1975, 14). The Catholic clergy played a direct role in locals, and strikes were viewed as a last resort. After losing many members to such organizations as the CIO, CLC, TLC, AFL, and the Federation Provincial du Travail (FPT) during the 1930s and 1940s, the CNTU became more secular and radical as a way of attracting membership. Strikes became more acceptable and widespread, and the CNTU came to be regarded as a threat to conservative forces in Quebec, including the Duplessis government (Rouillard 1981, 113, 167). By 1960, the organization's 442 locals had nearly 100,000 workers, about half the unionized workers in the province (Rouillard 1981, 167).

The CNTU had long represented workers from a wide range of industries, including pulp and paper, the service industry, clerical and office trades, the textile industry, metal trades, and mines. Local unions within these industry groups were organized into federations. Miners' unions had long been a component of the CNTU, and by 1960, the Mine Workers' Federation (MWF) had twelve unions with nearly 5,000 members (Rouillard 1981, 184). Despite this, the SLWPU was affiliated with the Metal Trades Federation (MTF), the same federation to which unions at Arvida and other Alcan aluminum plants (Shawinigan, Baie-Comeau, Lévis, and Beauharnois), and those at metal fabrication plants and foundries, were affiliated (Rouillard 1981, 245).

The likely rationale for affiliating the SLWPU to the MTF rather than the MWF was that many Quebec workers within the MTF were also employed by Alcan, and the Newfluor mine was directly linked to the Quebec aluminum industry. However, given the issues at stake in the St. Lawrence mines, the decision is questionable. Unions in the MWF, with their roots in the asbestos mining industry in such places as Asbestos, Thetford, and East Broughton, had a long history of health and safety struggles, including efforts in the 1940s to pressure the Quebec government into taking action on health hazards in the asbestos industry (Rouillard 1981, 132–33).

Despite any drawbacks that may have resulted from the MTF's lack of direct experience in the mining industry, however, the first collective agreement negotiated under the new affiliation contained some important gains for the SLWPU on the health and safety front. The 1963 agreement gave the union the right to have two designated members trained at company expense in the operation and reading of monitoring equipment and to have them participate in monitoring of radiation and dust at least every two weeks. The agreement also required that in cases where radiation or dust exceeded the safe working level, all workers were to be immediately removed from the affected area except those required to enter in order to remedy the hazard. According to the agreement, a safety committee with two company and two union representatives was to be established to conduct periodic tours of the underground and surface and to report potential hazards. The agreement also contained moderate wage increases.[55]

In addition to addressing health concerns through collective bargaining, the union continued to complain to government authorities about workplace conditions and practices. The Department of Mines was sometimes less than cooperative in dealing with these complaints. In April 1963, for instance, the Mines Minister gave what the union's solicitor described as a "truculent" reply to a number of complaints — implying that the company was responsible for ensuring that the mine regulations were enforced and that the union was outside its rights in demanding action on health and safety issues from his department.[56] When the Department of Mines insisted that "vague indictments" were not sufficient grounds for investigation, though, the union responded with a list of specific grievances: workers being disciplined for going to the lunch room for drinking water because all other water in the underground was contaminated by radiation; men working out of sight and sound of other workers; the union's ventilation monitor being pressured to concur with the company on radiation and dust readings; and the company interfering in the appointment of the union's monitor in order to get a man more friendly to the company's position.[57]

The union also charged that while the official lost-time injury rate at Newfluor was higher than that at Buchans mine and more than double that at the Bell Island (a fact borne out by the 1964 report of the Department of Mines, Agriculture and Resources), the actual rate was in fact higher because the company often neglected to report lost-time accidents in order to keep down its workers' compensation premiums. To the allegation that Newfluor had adopted this practice — commonly called "claims suppression" — the Mines Minister simply replied that the regulations required that all lost-time accidents be reported and that "the safety of workmen in the mines of St. Lawrence is of prime importance to my Department."[58]

The union continued to pressure the government, reporting in early 1964 that two men had recently been "gassed." The Department of Mines responded that it had not been informed of any such incident and that if it had occurred, the company was required to report it as a lost-time accident,

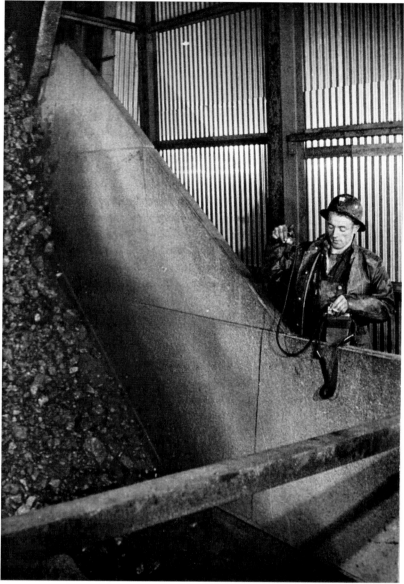

Miner Lawrence Edwards shines his light into an ore bin, c. 1965.

in which case it would appear in the Annual Report.[59] However, this was not entirely accurate, since an accident was only deemed "lost-time" if it prevented the worker from working on days beyond the day of the accident. This may explain why the alleged incident did not appear in the Annual Report (Department of Mines, Agriculture and Resources 1964, 171).

As the union persisted in its complaints about air quality and ventilation,

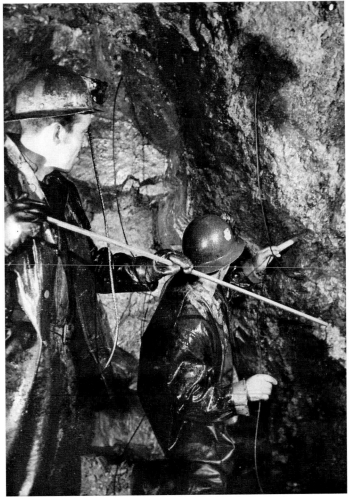

Loading blast holes with dynamite at the end of a shift, c. 1965.

the Department's responses grew more defensive and dismissive.[60] It defended the government's handling of the St. Lawrence situation and stated that until the union was willing to trust someone else's assessment and offer constructive criticism, its claims would not be considered or addressed.[61] The Department again demanded that the union make its complaints more specific and the union again responded with a list: that to cut costs the company shut down the ventilation system during weekends and holidays, so men returning after such breaks entered an atmosphere filled with "fumes, dust, and radiation"; that men were sent back into radiation-contaminated areas shortly after others had been taken out; that ventilation equipment was inadequate; and that blasting was carried out all through working hours.[62] The Department

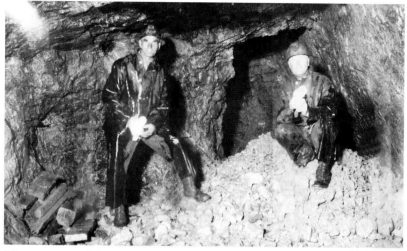

Miners atop an ore pile in a stope, c. 1965.

responded that it had spoken with the mine manager and been assured that there was no cause for concern and no need to issue further recommendations to the company.[63]

A review of the actual readings during this period reveals that the union had in fact good reason to be concerned about radiation levels. The company's monitoring reported at least three excessive readings during 1963, one of which showed a level nearly seven times the SWL. There were also several excessive readings during 1964, including one of more than four times the SWL, and seven during 1965, including three in July alone. The reports on these cases usually offered some explanation, such as damaged vent tubing or malfunctioning fans, and claimed that workers were removed from such areas as soon as the danger was discovered.[64] Company and government officials could also continue to claim that levels were within allowable limits because the final results of surveys were calculated as an average of the individual readings. The results for one week in 1965, for instance, show three readings in excess of the SWL, but the average of all the readings for that week was about half the SWL.[65] Periodic tests by the Chief Inspector showed similar results: on two occasions during 1964, the Inspector reported readings in excess of the SWL, but the average reading reported was only about one-third of the SWL.[66] For 1965, when at least seven readings were in excess of the SWL, the reported average was only about one-fifth of the SWL.[67] Since the results of individual tests were observed by a union representative every second week and the results forwarded to the union, excessive readings no doubt contributed to suspicion and controversy over this issue.

Antagonism between the union and the company was also apparently compounded by management's resentment of the CNTU's presence and influence. In 1965 Turpin noted that the Newfluor manager had asked him who was making the decisions in St. Lawrence, as it was management's understanding that it was the company and the union. Turpin replied that "we both have some higher ups looking after us."[68]

Though the SLWPU had apparently done well under Turpin's leadership during its affiliation with the CNTU, in 1966 the membership voted to replace him as president with Leo Slaney, a Newfluor employee for just three years at that point. The reasons for this decision are unclear; Turpin later claimed that he had come under criticism because his wife was being paid to clean and paint the union offices.[69] In any event, in April 1966, Slaney won the presidency by a very narrow margin, after which Turpin moved to Montreal, where he stayed for the remainder of his life.

Shortly after the change in union leadership, the Newfoundland government finally took a more active role in radiation monitoring, appointing a full-time monitor to take daily readings. This was quickly followed by Newfluor's hiring a safety officer whose duties included weekly monitoring of mine air.[70] Under the new system, both sets of readings were sent to Newfluor's Chief Engineer and to the union. Wiseman, the Newfluor manager, received the weekly average of these daily and weekly readings. The Department of Mines received these weekly averages every three months, except in instances when the reading was in excess of the SWL, which were to be reported to the Department immediately.[71] The new monitoring system apparently did little to ease tensions, however: asked later whether the introduction of daily readings improved relations between workers and the company, Wiseman simply replied, "Not that I've noticed."[72]

Notes

1. Turpin to C.W. Carter, M.P., House of Commons, Ottawa, 29 January 1958, MM.
2. Smallwood to Walter Seibert, 5 February 1958, Coll 075, File 3.20.087, CNSA.
3. A.H. Brown, Department of Labour, Ottawa, to Aloysius Turpin, SLWPU, 11 March 1958, MM; and Aloysius Turpin, SLWPU, to Michael Starr, Minister of Labour, Ottawa, 9 April 1958, MM.
4. Aloysius Turpin, SLWPU, to P.J. Lewis, 28 January 1958, MM.
5. Walter Seibert, St. Lawrence Corporation of Newfoundland, to Aloysius Turpin, SLWPU, 2 June 1957, Coll 079, File 7.39, CNSA.
6. Walter Seibert, St. Lawrence Corporation of Newfoundland, to Gordon Pushie, Director General of Economic Development, Province of Newfoundland, 3 November 1958, Coll 075, File 3.20.087, CNSA.
7. Gordon Pushie, Director General of Economic Development, Province of Newfoundland, to Joseph Smallwood, 3 November 1958, Coll 075, File 3.20.087, CNSA.
8. Aloysius Turpin, SLWPU, to P.J. Lewis, 10 February 1959, MM.

9. Aloysius Turpin, SLWPU, to Chairman of the Cancer Convention, St. John's, 28 January 1958, MM.

10. Leonard Miller to Dr. E.A. Watkinson, Chief of Occupational Health Division, National Health and Welfare, 30 June 1958, GN 78/1/B, 51 PANL; Leonard Miller to G.C. Brink, Director, Division of Tuberculosis Prevention, National Health and Welfare, 30 June 1958, GN 78/1/B, 51, PANL; and Leonard Miller to Dr. F.D. Brent, Chief Industrial Medical Officer, Alcan, Montreal, 30 June 1958, GN 78/1/B, 51, PANL.

11. Miller to Brink, 14 July 1958, GN 78/1/B, 51, PANL.

12. A.H. Sellers, Division of Medical Statistics, National Health and Welfare, to G.C. Brink, 25 July 1958, GN 78/1/B, 51, PANL; and G.C. Brink to Leonard Miller, 25 July 1958, GN 78/1/B, 51, PANL.

13. F.D. Brent, Alcan, to Miller, 18 July 1958, GN 78/1/B, 51, PANL.

14. Patterson to Miller, 2 April 1959, GN 78/1/B, 51, PANL.

15. Miller to Patterson, 16 July 1959, GN 78/1/B, 51, PANL.

16. Brent to Miller, 24 September 1959, GN 78/1/B, 51, PANL; and Turpin to C. Ballam, Minister of Labour, 23 November 1959, MM.

17. Aloysius Turpin, SLWPU, to James McGrath, Minster of Health, Government of Newfoundland, 30 June 1959, GN 78/1/B, 51, PANL.

18. James McGrath, Minister of Health, Government of Newfoundland, to Turpin, 4 March 1960, MM.

19. Brent to McGrath, 22 January 1960, GN 78/1/B, 51, PANL.

20. W.J. Keough, Minister of Mines, to McGrath, 3 March 1960, GN 78/1/B, 51. PANL.

21. Canada, Department of Labour, RG27, Vol. 540, Reel T-3401, Strike 39, NAC.

22. Turpin to Smallwood, 12 March 1960, Coll 075, File 3.20.087, CNSA.

23. Donald Poynter, St. Lawrence Fluorspar/St. Lawrence Corporation, to N.S. Batten, Unemployment Insurance Commission, St. John's, 28 March 1960, RG27, Vol. 540, Reel T-3401, Strike 39, NAC.

24. Keough to McGrath, 23 March 1960, GN 78/1/B, 51, PANL.

25. Wiseman to Gover, 25 March 1960, GN 78/1/B, 51, PANL.

26. J.P. Windish, Department of National Health and Welfare, Occupational Health Division, to St. Lawrence Workers' Protective Union, 3 April 1960, GN 78/1/B, 51, PANL.

27. Labour Canada, Report on Industrial Dispute Termination: Dispute between St. Lawrence Corporation of Newfoundland, Newfoundland Fluorspar Limited, and St. Lawrence Workers' Protective Union, RG27, Vol. 540, Reel T-3401, Strike 39, NAC.

28. Poynter to Batten, Unemployment Insurance Commission, 4 May 1960, RG27, Vol. 540, Reel T-3401, Strike 39, NAC.

29. Howard Farrell, Report of the Mining Properties of St. Lawrence Corporation, 1967, 40–54, File 1L/14, DME.

30. Turpin to B.J. Trevor, Chief Inspector of Mines, Department of Mines and Resources, 18 May 1960, MM.

31. Windish to Miller, 28 July 1960, GN 78/1/B, 51, PANL.

32. Miller to Trevor, 27 July 1960, GN 78/1/B, 51, PANL.

33. McGrath to Keough, 29 March 1960 GN 78/1/B, 51, PANL.
34. Turpin to Lewis, 21 September 1960, MM.
35. Turpin to Lewis, 21 September 1960, MM.
36. Canada, Labour Canada, Report on Industrial Dispute Commencement, RG 27, Vol. 543, Reel T3402, Strike 202, NAC.
37. Statement of R. Wisemen, General Manager, Newfoundland Fluorspar Company, St. Lawrence, 27 October 1960, RG 27, Vol. 543, Reel T3402, Strike 202, NAC.
38. Canada, Labour Canada, Report on Industrial Dispute Termination, RG 27, Vol. 543, Reel T3402, Strike 202, NAC.
39. Miller to Gover, 27 July 1960, GN 78/1/B, 51, PANL.
40. St. Lawrence Corporation of Newfoundland, List of Employees From Whom Union Dues Were Collected for the Month of January 1961, MM.
41. St. Lawrence Corporation of Newfoundland, List of Employees From Whom Union Dues Were Collected for the Month of July 1961, and For the Month of November 1961, MM.
42. Lukins, Chief Inspector of Mines, to R. Wiseman, Newfluor, 30 January 1961, MM.
43. Lukins to Newfoundland Department of Mines and Resources, 3 April 1961, GN 78/1/B, 51, PANL; and Lukins to Deputy Minister of Mines, 2 May 1962, GN 78/1/B, 51, PANL.
44. Keough to Turpin, 30 November 1961, MM.
45. Interview with Richard Loder, 15 October 2000.
46. Lukins to Deputy Minister of Mines, 2 May 1962, GN 78/1/B, 51, PANL.
47. McGrath to Father Hogan, Parish Priest, St. Lawrence, 5 April 1962; and McGrath to P.J. Lewis, 5 April 1962, GN 78/1/B, 51, PANL.
48. Lukins to Deputy Minister of Mines, 2 May 1962, GN 78/1/B, 51, PANL.
49. Canada, Labour Canada, Report on Industrial Dispute Commencement, RG 27, Vol. 550, Reel T3405, Strike 23, NAC.
50. Canada, Labour Canada, Report on Industrial Dispute Termination, RG 27, Vol. 550, Reel T3405, Strike 23, NAC.
51. Research Associates Limited, Montreal, to Turpin, 27 June 1959, MM.
52. International Union of Mine, Mill and Smelter Workers, Toronto, to Turpin, 25 February 1960, MM.
53. Extract of the Minutes of a Special General Meeting of the St. Lawrence Workers' Protective Union held on 29 October 1962, MM.
54. Ted Payne, Vice-President, CNTU, to Turpin, 8 November 1962, MM.
55. Collective Agreement between Newfoundland Fluorspar Limited and St. Lawrence Workers' Protective Union, 9 March 1963, AA.
56. Lewis to Turpin, 11 April 1963, MM.
57. Turpin to W.J. Keough, Minister, Mines, Agriculture, and Resources: Union Report with Regards to the Fluorspar Industry Operated by the Newfoundland Fluorspar Company, 16 April 1963, MM.
58. Keough to Carter, 26 August 1963, and forwarded to Turpin, 20 September 1963, MM.
59. Carter to Turpin, 15 January 1964, re: reply from Keough to Carter, 10 January 1964, MM.

60. Turpin to C.H. Ballam, Minister of Labour, Government of Newfoundland, 11 March 1964, MM.
61. Keough to Lewis, 24 March 1964, MM.
62. For example: Turpin to Lewis, 31 March 1964, MM.
63. Lewis to Turpin, 26 May 1964, re: Deputy Minister of Mines to Lewis, 14 May 1964, and Brian J. Trevor, Chief Inspector of Mines, to Keough, 28 May 1964, MM.
64. Results of Mine Ventilation Surveys Conducted by Newfoundland Fluorspar Limited, 1963, 1964, and 1965, MM.
65. Results of Mine Ventilation Surveys Conducted by Newfoundland Fluorspar Limited, 21–25 July 1965, MM.
66. Trevor to Keough, 15 June 1964, and 23 November 1964, MM.
67. Survey Lung Cancer of St. Lawrence Miners, GN78/1/B, 220, File 290/G/07, PANL.
68. Turpin to Adrian Proude, Secretary, MTF, 9 March 1965, MM.
69. Interview with Aloysius Turpin, MUNFLA.
70. GN 6, 2, PANL.
71. GN 6, 2, PANL.
72. GN 6, 2, PANL.

Chapter Five

"THE TRULY GHASTLY TOTAL" AND THE LACK OF COMPENSATION COVERAGE

The Toll Taken and the Rennie Slaney Submission

Findings on radiation levels sparked ongoing disputes over workplace hazards and how they were being dealt with. The period following these findings was also marked by further confirmation of the death toll up to that time, a continuation of rampant disease and mortality, and a more intense focus on the matter of compensation for victims and their dependents. A federal study concluded that from 1933 to 1961, among employees of both companies, twenty-two had died from silicosis or silico-tuberculosis, twenty-six from lung cancer, seventeen from other cancers, twenty-one from circulatory system diseases, twenty-nine from other known causes, and four from unknown causes. The average age of death for lung cancer victims was forty-seven years, with the youngest victim up to that point thirty-three years old and the oldest fifty-six. The average length of underground exposure for lung cancer victims was just over twelve years, the average time from first exposure to death nineteen years, and the average time from last exposure to death just under two years (de Villiers and Windish 1964).

The study also concluded that death from lung cancer among St. Lawrence miners was more frequent than even some of the most notorious cases documented up to that time. For example, the average age at death from lung cancer among St. Lawrence miners was lower than that among uranium miners in Germany and Czechoslovakia in the late 1800s, and the average time from first exposure to death was shorter. The percentage of lung cancer deaths at St. Lawrence was much higher than that among uranium miners in South Africa, and the average age of death was about ten years younger (de Villiers and Windish 1964). Looking at the health status of the 280 men employed at the mines in 1960 and of nearly a hundred former miners, the study concluded beyond a doubt that exposure to radiation was the cause of the high incidence of lung cancer among miners (Bartlett et al. 1964). By 1963, six more miners had died from cancer of the lung and respiratory system, bringing the total to thirty-two (de Villiers 1966). In 1965, it was confirmed that forty-one others were suffering from lung cancer and that victims were dying at a younger age.[1]

This rate of disease and death naturally drew increased attention to the matter of compensation for victims and their dependents. In direct response to the St. Lawrence situation, lung cancer caused by exposure to radiation was included under workers' compensation coverage in July 1960 (Newfoundland 1961). At that time, WCB Chairman Irving Fogwill suggested that the cost of pending and future claims arising out of St. Lawrence could be "staggering." Therefore, it was decided that the benefits paid for St. Lawrence claims would not come out of the regular Accident Fund into which mine operators paid their premiums but out of the Disaster Reserve Fund, into which a portion of premiums from all employers was directed.[2] One effect of this decision was to absolve employers at St. Lawrence of their financial liability for cancer claims. The decision also undermined the basic principle of the workers' compensation system: that tying premium levels to claim levels motivates employers to provide a safe and healthy workplace. In fact, Newfluor manager Wiseman later stated that once his company was assured that claims would be paid out of the Disaster Fund and therefore not affect the company's premium levels, it abandoned its policy of refusing to hire former St. Lawrence Corporation workers: Newfluor would now not be financially liable in the event that they developed an industrial disease.[3]

The limit on the scope of coverage and on the retroactivity of the Act also continued to bar many from actually accessing compensation benefits. The 1960 amendment extended coverage only to cases of lung cancer, and as with coverage for silicosis, did not apply to cases where the worker left the job before the Act came into effect in April 1951. These provisions had a real, detrimental effect on the lives of miners and their families, as illustrated by just a few examples. In one case, a miner had worked underground at Newfluor from 1947 to 1961, when he was forced to quit because of "shortness of breath." His compensation claim was denied because his ailment was not covered by the Act, leaving him, his wife, and five children to live on social assistance. Another worked at Newfluor from 1948 to 1960 and was told that he would not be compensated for his chronic obstructive lung disease as he had neither cancer nor silicosis. He was told to do "light work," but lacking education, could find no such work.[4] In another case, a miner worked with both companies for seventeen years and continued working until two weeks before he died of cancer in 1949, at the age of thirty-nine. His wife died three months later. The compensation claim was denied because he died two years before the Act came into effect. Instead, his son worked to raise his seven brothers and sisters with some help from the grandfather.[5] A miner who had worked for the St. Lawrence Corporation died of lung cancer in 1944, leaving his wife and nine children, aged nine days to sixteen years at the time, to survive on social assistance. An Iron Springs miner died in 1945 at the age of twenty-seven, leaving his wife to raise their two children on social assistance. Another St. Lawrence Corporation miner was just twenty-three years old when shortness of breath forced him to leave work in 1945. He was sent to the tuberculosis sanitarium but his illness was never conclusively diagnosed. When he died two years later at the age of twenty-five, his widow was denied compensation because of the inconclusive diagnosis and the year of his death. Another miner worked underground for the St. Lawrence Corporation until forced to quit in 1949 because of an illness later diagnosed as lung cancer. Because he had left work two years before the Act came into effect, he, his wife, and five children had to live on social assistance.

The plight faced by former workers is starkly illustrated by a letter to one claimant in 1960, in which the WCB expressed confusion that the man did not appear relieved when his x-ray showed no silicosis. For men in his situation, however, a disease that qualified for compensation was the only hope for some level of income support. In other cases, claims were denied because the person had not worked underground. For example, one man who worked in the St. Lawrence Corporation's processing mill in the 1930s and 1940s developed what appeared to be silicosis and then lung cancer. He died in 1964, but the claim was denied because he had only worked on the surface. In another case, when a surface worker at Newfluor died of lung cancer in 1955, the WCB denied the widow's claim on the same grounds.[6]

While those affected struggled daily with industrial disease and a lack of support, the issue began to gain wider attention only in 1965, when it was brought to the notice of a committee appointed to review the Workmen's Compensation Act. Among the submissions received by the committee, there was one it described as so "extraordinary" and "startling" that it demanded special attention. The brief was submitted by Rennie Slaney, a former St. Lawrence Corporation employee and a witness to the Issac Slaney autopsy in 1952. Slaney's brief described working conditions from the start of mining in St. Lawrence and the effects of industrial disease on miners and their families. His submission also listed the names of eighty-four dead miners, more than seventy of whom he claimed had died from lung cancer and respiratory diseases. Slaney also claimed that in only about twenty-five of these seventy cases had dependents received any compensation. He also listed thirteen cases of former miners too sick from cancer and respiratory diseases to work, only six of whom were being compensated (Winter 1966, 42–49).

While conceding that these figures were unofficial, the Review Committee nonetheless accepted them as "fairly reliable," given Slaney's first-hand knowledge of the subject. However, information the Review Committee got from the WCB was quite different. The WCB identified 1952 as the year of the first recorded death from industrial disease associated with the St. Lawrence mines, and claimed that from then until 1965 there were thirty-four deaths from lung cancer in St. Lawrence miners, as well as four deaths from silicosis and silico-tuberculosis. In addition, the WCB's records showed just seven cases of silicotic miners still living, with varying degrees of disability. The Review Committee attributed the discrepancy to the simple fact that some cases had not been compensated and therefore were not captured in the WCB statistics. The Committee concluded that the figures provided by Slaney were "much nearer the truly ghastly total than the fifty-odd in the Board's files" (Winter 1966, 50).

The Review Committee recommended a thorough investigation of the St. Lawrence situation to uncover not only the medical and scientific dimensions of the case but also "the sociological and human side of the tragedy, the tale of which has been only partially and superficially told" (Winter 1966, 51). Forced to take action by the sheer magnitude of the problem and the decisive conclusions of the Review Committee, the Newfoundland Government announced in February 1967 the appointment of a Royal Commission to investigate industrial disease and workers' compensation at St. Lawrence.

Clean Skirts and Death Traps: The PR Battle Heats Up

The release of the Review Committee's report and the establishment of the Royal Commission intensified both internal and public debate over the handling of the St. Lawrence situation. For example, Premier Smallwood himself criticized a newspaper article that used the Review Committee's phrase "national disaster" to describe the situation (*Evening Telegram* March 31, 1967). A Health Department official pointed to the article as an example of how the situation had been "blown out of proportion," and complained that for all the publicity given to St. Lawrence no one had mentioned the "vast sums of money pumped into the St. Lawrence mines project" by the Newfoundland government.[7] It is unclear exactly what money this referred to. Smallwood criticized media coverage of the St. Lawrence case as "greatly exaggerated" and dismissed much of it as "history."[8]

Newfluor also entered this latest battle in the war of words. In a press release purporting to present a more balanced view than that offered by the media, the company complained that the publicity had been "very much one-sided, with the grim side of the picture being highlighted and exaggerated and the brighter side of the picture being entirely eliminated," leaving the public "grossly misinformed." The release attempted to counter the negative publicity by describing the economic benefits the mining industry had brought to the town and defending Newfluor's health and safety record.[9] But the "grim side of the picture" continued to be displayed in such forms as a television special exploring the history of mining and industrial disease in the community and a scathing newspaper article by Rennie Slaney describing the history of working conditions, the toll taken on the people, and the government's mishandling of the matter (*Evening Telegram* March 31, 1967).

The public controversy was intensified by a major accident in September 1967, when a fall of rock on the 550-foot level of Director mine killed three miners. Rescue crews took several days to recover the bodies, buried under several tons of rock (Newfoundland Department of Mines, Agriculture and Resources 1968, 222–40). The union and community residents were outraged by the triple fatality, which sparked another storm of controversy in the press. In a St. John's newspaper article describing Director as the "Killer Mine," the union president stated that the men had feared that area for some time as it had been the site of frequent "rockbursts" — the sudden shifting of rock that triggered the 1967 collapse — and many narrow escapes. (*Evening Telegram* September 18, 1967). Indeed, rockbursting had been a concern at Director since at least 1959, when the company began studying the problem,[10] and the union as well as individual workers became increasingly concerned about the problem during the 1960s.[11] Jerome Spearns recalled an incident from the mid-1960s when he and several others escaped danger when they heard the noise that often preceded rockbursting and left the area over the protests of the supervisor. Though a veteran miner at the time, Spearns was plagued by fears and could not sleep at night; rockbursting at Director became so bad that in 1966, he and several others left St. Lawrence for a recently opened copper mine in northeastern Newfoundland.[12]

Activist Rennie Slaney noted that the accident had added three more to the death toll, bringing to twenty-seven the number of men who had lived within a 250-foot radius of his house and been killed by industrial diseases or accidents (*Evening Telegram* September 18, 1967). Several St. Lawrence miners quit their jobs immediately after the accident, and Newfluor workers refused to report for work for the day following the funerals. According to the union president, many men now went underground believing that "they are going to their doom," and one former miner suffering from lung cancer remarked, "That death trap ought to be closed and never allowed to be opened again" (*Evening Telegram* September 19, 1967). Because the most recent victims had left a total of eighteen dependents, the accident also drew public attention to the plight of the widows and children in St. Lawrence. One woman described having lived for ten years on welfare in a "two room shack," while another spoke of watching her husband die of cancer "while nine children gather at your back waiting to be fed" (*Evening Telegram* September 19, 1967).

Newfluor management responded to the most recent outpouring of negative publicity by again trying to correct what it called "inaccuracies" in the media's coverage. Wiseman pointed out that seven miners had been killed by accidents over the entire life of the Director mine (*Evening Telegram* September 29, 1967). He did not mention the number killed by industrial diseases. Wiseman also disputed recent claims that the company was having difficulty getting St. Lawrence men to work underground because of health

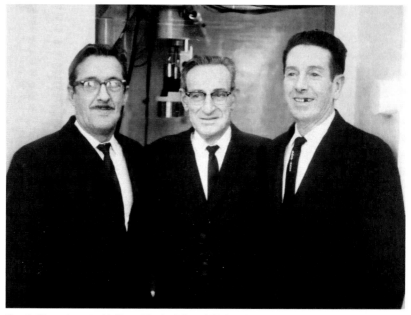

Rennie Slaney (centre) with Harry Turpin (left) and Clyde Lake (right), a delegation that visited Ottawa in connection with the Royal Commission, c. 1967. Slaney died shortly after the release of the report.

and safety concerns (*Evening Telegram* September 29, 1967).

A key element in Newfluor's public relations efforts was the 1968 establishment of a newsletter called the *Newfluor News*. This publication served a variety of purposes — it advertised local events, provided sports and other community news, and served as a forum for local service organizations. It was also used to put a good face on Newfluor's safety record and its contribution to the community. The March 1968 issue, for example, contained an article about a piece published in the magazine *Canadian Scientist* stating that ventilation and monitoring had rendered Director mine free of radiation hazards, as well as an article summarizing Newfluor's handling of the rockburst problem at Director (*Newfluor News* March, 1968, 1–2). An October 1968 article on a recent visit of the "Alcan Medical Team" to St. Lawrence included subheadings such as "Employees Express Satisfaction," and "Doctors Impressed" (*Newfluor News* October 1968, 1). The Alcan Medical Team, which began visiting St. Lawrence annually in early 1968, was itself part of the public relations campaign, established, according to Dr. Brent, to give St. Lawrence "the kind of Company health program that is available to Alcan employees in other parts of Canada" (*Newfluor News* October 1968, 1). The company began to hand out Safety Medallions to employees who had gone a certain number of hours without a lost-time accident, instituted a "Twenty-Five Year Club" to honour workers achieving that length of service, and established a "Wise Owl Club" to recognize workers who protected their health and safety (*Newfluor News* November 1968, 1). The *Newfluor News* was also used as a forum for publishing average radiation readings and anything else that contributed to polishing the company's image.

As well, Newfluor began using community organizations as part of its public relations campaign. Wiseman helped found a community service organization called the Lion's Club, in which Safety Officer Gerry Drover and other staff members were key figures. In 1968, Newfluor began sponsoring an annual Christmas event where children of current or former Newfluor employees received a gift from "Santa Claus." The company continued at the same time to operate through more private channels to win the support of government officials. In May 1968, for instance, Harry Ethridge of Alcan's Public Relations Department sent provincial Health Minister John C. Crosbie a magazine article entitled "Alcan Companies Play Major Role in Eradicating Miners' Sickness."[13]

In March 1968, the company brought in additional professional help for its public relations campaign. Eric Trist, an expert in "Organizational Theory" from the University of California, was brought to St. Lawrence for one week to conduct a field study in the community and provide recommendations on improving community morale and labour relations. Trist claimed that a lot of anxiety about the radiation hazard lingered among those not actually employed in the mines, such as the "wives and mothers of those likely to be exposed" and people outside the community, but that most of those actually working underground believed the mine to be safe.

Trist commended management for what he considered good public relations moves such as a recent decision to post daily radiation readings. According to Trist, the establishment of the *Newfluor News*, the formation of the Alcan Medical Team, and the introduction of a company-sponsored weekly radio broadcast called "St. Lawrence Report" had done much to "communicate a more rational understanding" of the situation and to project a more positive image of the company. The *Newfluor News*, in his assessment, was especially effective, since "Anything it says about radiation is the more readily believed because the facts it reports about community activities can be verified by the readers." He recommended that the company continue and extend such efforts, make more use of community groups such as the Lion's Club, and contribute substantially to a fund being proposed for the construction of a recreational facility (Trist 1968, 2–49).

On a negative note, Trist claimed that any trust that existed was "brittle," citing as evidence the union's claim that if and when the government's daily radiation monitor left St. Lawrence, the company would not conduct the daily readings because it simply would not be willing to pay a man to do it. He suggested that a major contributor to the morale problem plaguing the workplace and the community was the fact that supervisory staff were almost invariably from mainland Canada or Europe; the lack of local men in these positions contributed to social differentiation and resentment (Trist 1968, 16–17).

Trist also noted that health and safety problems at the mines had eroded the sense of self-worth among the underground workforce and given rise to the belief among young men that the mine was where you might be forced to go if you did not do well in school (Trist 1968, 16–17). He touched upon the dilemma in which workers in such situations often found themselves. Closure of sections of Director mine after the accident of September 1967 had resulted in about fifty men being put out of work while repairs were being made. Trist stated that the men were torn between their belief that the Director mine was dangerous and their desire to get the mine back into full production and return to work (Trist 1968, 10–13).

Newfluor management questioned a number of Trist's suggestions, including his recommendation that the company assume responsibility for daily radiation readings should the government withdraw that service, since in the company's view, these readings were unnecessary. However, management agreed with other propositions. One of these was that efforts be made to get the union president to become a paid employee of the company rather than of the union, and that he then be involved in radiation readings and other health and safety measures, something Trist claimed the union president favoured. The company believed this would have the combined effect of giving the president's stamp of approval to health and safety matters and familiarizing him with the daily operations of the mine. Management also agreed that the company should continue and increase its public relations efforts.[14]

The Royal Commission

Trist had also noted that a "favourable" report from the Royal Commission would be most likely to instill confidence among workers and the general public. However, given the union's continuing complaints over radiation and other hazards, deep grievances over deaths, disease, and the lack of compensation coverage, and the recent triple fatality, it is not surprising that the atmosphere of the Royal Commission's first public session in St. Lawrence in November 1967 was charged.

The Royal Commission was chaired by lawyer Fintan Aylward, the son of Patrick Aylward, the local businessman who had started the first union in 1939. The Aylward family had steadily risen to prominence through their business ventures in St. Lawrence and across the province. By 1967, their St. Lawrence businesses included a supermarket, building supplies store, service station, and real estate, as well as a bar, the Laurentian Club, which was the center of social life for many miners. His selection as chair may have been based on the Aylward family's allegiance to the Liberal Party, but if the Smallwood government had expected Fintan Aylward to produce a report that suited their needs, they were to be unpleasantly surprised. The other members of the Commission were Dr. Bliss Murphy, a prominent Newfoundland radiologist, Frederick Gover, Deputy Minister of Mines and former Chief Inspector, and Dr. David Parsons, who had assisted in the earlier studies on cancer among the miners.[15] The Commission's terms of reference included investigating all compensation claims made by any miner or miner's dependent; determining the number of dependents not receiving compensation in cases where the husband or father had apparently died of lung cancer or any possible work-related disease since the start of mining; and investigating the WCB's handling of claims from miners and their dependents (Newfoundland March 7, 1967).

The session was taken up primarily with the Newfluor submission. Company representatives defended Newfluor's safety record and claimed that the company had always cooperated with government and medical officials in detecting and responding to health hazards. They also expressed the hope that the Royal Commission would "inspire confidence among the present Newfluor work force and all members of the general public in Newfoundland that working conditions in Director mine are not a hazard to health today and have not constituted a hazard to the health of fluorspar miners for the past seven years."[16]

Newfluor representatives suggested that negative distortion of the St. Lawrence situation had caused a shortage of skilled miners and led to production problems. The company noted that of seventy underground miners employed by Newfluor in 1959, only seventeen remained on the payroll in 1967.[17] While there was no further analysis of these figures, it is safe to assume that a portion of what Newfluor called the "exodus of local experienced miners" was an exodus to the local hospitals and cemeteries.

Based on its interpretation of the situation, the company submitted four recommendations: that a third doctor be stationed in the community; that a single radiologist be put in charge of analyzing chest x-rays of St. Lawrence miners; that the Workmen's Compensation Act be amended to remove the limit on the time a worker suffering from an industrial disease had from cessation of employment to the filing of a claim; and that a "Special Fund" be established to provide financial assistance to former miners incapacitated prior to 1967 or to their dependents, in cases where it could be shown that workers' compensation and other forms of support were not adequate.[18] Significantly, none of these recommendations committed the company to bearing any specific or substantial cost for the tragedy.

Discussion of the company's presentation provided important insights into its handling of the situation. For instance, Wiseman revealed that the company had conducted tests for radiation at Director mine as early as 1952, but had found no significant levels. Wiseman stated that these tests were prompted by the discovery of valuable uranium deposits in Ontario and that the company had checked the mine out of "curiosity."[19] He also stated that when the 1959–60 tests revealed high levels of radiation at Director mine and at the St. Lawrence Corporation mines, the company assumed that the testing instrument used in 1952 had been malfunctioning.[20]

Union president Leo Slaney attended the session but no CNTU representative was present, despite assurances given to Slaney that one would attend.[21] Slaney challenged Wiseman to explain why, when the company had been told by Windish in November 1959 that there were dangerous levels of radiation at Director mine, the men not been informed of this and had been permitted to continue working there until March 1960. Slaney also disputed Wiseman's claim that no work was done in the most contaminated area, the 550-foot level, after the discovery of radiation, until additional ventilation was installed there.[22] Before Wiseman could respond to these challenges, the chair advised Slaney that he and the union would have the opportunity to speak at the end of the session or to present a brief so that "both sides" of the story could be heard. At this point, James Cameron, Alcan's Managing Director, who had been brought in from Montreal for the hearing, objected to use of the term "both sides." "I think we are striving for the facts here," Cameron insisted, "there is no such thing as 'both sides'."[23] Several times during the proceedings, Cameron, Wiseman, and Frank Brent insisted that the company had taken adequate steps to deal with the problem based on the information available to it at the time. Brent declared that "we wanted to do everything we could to keep the Company's skirts as clean as possible."[24]

Wiseman also stated that of the three government inspectors who periodically visited St. Lawrence, two had never entered the underground.[25] Regarding the procedure for dealing with a radiation-contaminated area, asked whether it was sealed off from the other working areas in any way to limit the movement of radon gas through the mine, Wiseman stated that such areas were simply blocked from access by a couple of boards.[26] Newfluor Safety Officer Gerry Drover was asked by a commissioner whether he had ever received any instructions about where to position the instrument when taking a radiation test, to which he replied no.[27] Drover was also asked whether he could sense when the radiation reading in a particular area might be high, to which he replied, "I can't, but some of the miners claim they can." He also stated that the miners were very interested in the radiation readings and asked him about it "all the time."[28]

The Royal Commission's second public hearing was scheduled for May 1968, in St. Lawrence, and Leo Slaney was determined to have the CNTU help prepare the union's submission. Slaney wrote directly to CNTU President Marcel Pepin to complain that the submission was not ready, and Commission Chair Aylward wrote to CNTU General Secretary Robert Sauvé reminding him of an earlier promise to get the submission in.[29] There are several possible reasons for the delay. Ted Payne, who had been acting as advisor to the SLWPU on behalf of the CNTU since affiliation in 1963, was ill and off the job during the fall and winter of 1967–68.[30] At the administrative level, the Mines Federation and the Metal Trades Federation were going through a complex process of amalgamation at the time (Rouillard 1981, 258–60). Moreover, the Quiet Revolution and increasing political unrest in Quebec were bringing new pressures to bear on organizations such as the CNTU in this period, and the CNTU was being drawn into the political upheaval sweeping the province (Güntzel 2000; Rouillard 1981, 369–96). In short, factors within the CNTU and within Quebec were not conducive to giving prompt attention to the St. Lawrence union and the Royal Commission.

Payne was back on the St. Lawrence case in January 1968, but there are indications that he was not very familiar with the issues being considered by the Royal Commission: Slaney had to explain to him in very simple terms what a rockburst was and what dangers it presented, as well as what the radiation hazard consisted of and the methods for dealing with it.[31] Payne's lack of knowledge in these areas is not surprising, for he had had limited involvement with occupational health and safety issues despite having been the SLWPU's Technical Advisor for five years. The fact that Payne was from the Metal Workers' Federation, not the Miners' Federation, no doubt limited his knowledge of these areas.

Despite the limitations, the union's submission was ready in time for the May 1968 hearing, and Payne was in attendance to help present it. The union charged that both the historical and current conditions at the mines were evidence that the company was "unable or unwilling to apply control measures" and that this indicated the need for increased government intervention.[32] Summarizing the history of mining and industrial disease in St. Lawrence, the union claimed that the bitterness and mistrust harboured by workers and others arose not from a lack of understanding of the facts, but the opposite: it arose from the knowledge that so many had died and would die a horrible and unnecessary death for the sake of "industrial development and corporate profits." The union also pointed out that, having paid this "terrible price," many had been left unable to care for themselves and their families.[33]

The union made several recommendations to improve conditions at the mines. These included increased ventilation and monitoring and the establishment of a pro-active health and safety program to replace the "trial and error" method used in the past. It recommended that the scope of workers' compensation coverage be broadened and benefits increased, and requested compensation for all claims dating back to 1933.[34]

The third and final public hearing, held in St. Lawrence in April 1969, dealt primarily with the submission of the St. Lawrence Town Council. Though brief, the Town Council's submission was direct and highly critical, especially of the provincial government:

> Rigid and proper inspection in the mines would have reduced sub-stantially the hazardous conditions prevailing in the stopes long be-fore this [ventilation and monitoring] system was introduced.... The time has come when procrastination on the part of all Departments of Government must be frowned upon, condemned and proscribed by those responsible.[35]

The Town Council argued that most improvements in working conditions at the mines over the years had been brought about not out of concern and proactive efforts by the government or employers but by "persistent and insistent demands for intervention, regulation and control by Union leaders and respectable citizens."[36] The Council submission pressed the need for alternate industries in a context where dependence on a single industry left the people "particularly susceptible to the hazards associated with industrial activity."[37]

In addition to holding these public hearings, the Royal Commission also investigated mortality and disease rates, workers' compensation claims, and the plight of disabled miners and dependents. From 1933 to 1967, it discovered, fifty-three miners had died from cancer of lungs and trachea, twenty-five from silicosis and silico-tuberculosis, nine from other diseases of the respiratory system, twenty-one from cancer of the stomach and digestive system, ten from other cancers, and sixty-one from diseases of the heart and cardiovascular system. Of the fifty-three deaths from cancer of the trachea and lungs, thirty-five of the victims had been under fifty-five years old, and twenty-four had died in just four years, from 1963 to 1967 (Aylward 1969, 178–79).

The Commission drew special attention to cancer of the stomach and digestive system, which accounted for two-thirds of all other cancer deaths among miners. While the rate of death from this cause was roughly the same among surface and underground employees, there was a striking dif-ference in the average age of death: for surface workers with this type of cancer, the average age of death was just over seventy-one years, while for underground workers, it was just under fifty-three years. The report noted that the discrepancy "may be suggestive of an as yet unrecognized aspect of occupational exposure" related to drinking the water in mines and from the town's public water supplies. In fact, the public supplies had been tested as part of the radiation studies conducted in 1959–60 and found to contain much higher than normal levels of radon-222 (Aylward 1969, 136–37). The Commission suggested that this might explain the fact that the average age at death from stomach cancer was lower in St. Lawrence than in neighbouring communities. Alternate public supplies had been established after the 1959–60 findings and the Commission suggested that these be monitored regularly for radon levels (Aylward 1969, 134). There is no evidence that this was ever done.

The Commission also met with individuals to assess the effects of industrial disease and the application of the Workmen's Compensation Act on miners and their families over the years. In addition to many cases of the kind already described, where benefits had been denied for various reasons, the Commission found several other features of the system that had detrimental outcomes for victims and their families. For example, in cases of "partial disability," benefits were based on the degree of disability, the implication being that such workers could continue to earn wages to supplement their compensation benefits. This bore little relation to reality as many workers — physically incapacitated, lacking education and other skills, and living in what was essentially a single-industry town — simply could not do so. The union's submission had cited an example of one former miner who had taken up fishing to supplement his benefits and was so incapacitated he had to be helped from his boat onto the wharf by a rope.[38]

The Royal Commission also found that benefits were woefully inadequate. In 1969, the widow of a deceased miner received, upon her husband's death, a $300 lump sum and thereafter $100 per month for herself and $35 per month for each dependent child. However, the maximum amount of compensation payable per month, in cases of both disability and death, regardless of the number of dependents, was $312.50. In a community where large families were the norm, this left many in dire circumstances.[39]

Another serious problem arose from fact that while there had been moderate increases in benefits since 1951, the level of benefit actually paid in individual cases continued to be based on the amount in effect at the time of disablement or death. Thus recipients did not receive any increases in benefits introduced since their claim had been accepted. This not only left payments abysmally low and out of step with the increased cost of living in many cases, but also created differences in the amounts received. The Commission found this to be a major complaint of the widows interviewed, so much so that it urged the WCB to address the problem immediately. An amendment passed in July 1967 accordingly made all widows eligible for rates then in effect (Aylward 1969, 233–34).

The Commission discovered many instances where widows had no indoor plumbing, could not carry out basic maintenance on their homes, and were unable to provide decent winter clothing for their children.[40] Widows receiving compensation benefits, especially those with large families, were in many cases worse off financially than those on social assistance (Aylward 1969, 232–33). Many of these women had no access to other means of support and could hardly turn to their family or neighbours for help when so many in the community were in the same position. The Commission concluded that it was "unjust, humiliating and degrading for widows of deceased workmen who died as a result of an occupational disease" to be left in this position (Aylward 1969, 260–61).

In assessing the WCB's justification for rejecting these claims, the Commission questioned the adequacy of the legislation but concluded that the WCB had been "reasonably efficient in handling the majority of the claims" within its legislative boundaries. (Aylward 1969, 266). However, while WCB staff may have been efficient, they were sometimes less than professional. For example, in one instance, a WCB medical officer wrote to a claimant who had worked underground for twenty years that, "I think the impression in St. Lawrence is that all ailments, infections, allergies, etc., will be covered by the Board."[41]

The Commission also identified neglected opportunities to have dealt more adequately with the disaster and with the culpability of some parties. It noted that the union's appeal for x-rays in 1942 had been "a reasonable request" and that it was "indeed most unfortunate" that it had not been granted. The Commission also criticized the St. Lawrence Corporation's handling of industrial disease, noting that even after official diagnosis of the first silicosis case in 1952, the St. Lawrence Corporation manager "refused to believe that silicosis was present" (Aylward 1969, 164). There was little discussion of the role played by the Department of Mines, but the Commission did criticize the provincial Department of Heath for being "slow in its acknowledgment of serious occupational health hazards in the mines" and the federal Department of Health and Welfare for being "unwarrantedly bureaucratic" in its response to the situation in the 1950s (Aylward 1969, 34, 42). This was a reference to the federal Department's response to Pepper's request in 1950 that it investigate the possible link between working conditions and disease among miners at St. Lawrence, when it stated that it would act on such a request only if it came from the provincial Department of Health. This inaction contributed to delaying federal involvement until 1957.

The Commission's final report, submitted to government in July 1969, contained sixty-nine recommendations, the most important of which were: that since the cause of various pulmonary diseases (such as bronchitis, silicosis, tuberculosis and tumors) was often complex and indeterminate, loss of pulmonary function be taken into account when considering any compensation claim; that the dependents of every miner who had died or would die from lung cancer or silicosis receive compensation regardless of the date of death; that anyone disabled by lung cancer or silicosis at any time be compensated; that coverage be extended to cases of tuberculosis, any chronic obstructive pulmonary disease, and cancers other than lung cancers, such as cancer of the nose or throat; that a "Special Fund" be established with contributions from employers and the provincial and federal governments to augment compensation benefits where appropriate; that the monthly ceiling on benefits to widows be eliminated; and that a second government radiation monitor be stationed at St. Lawrence (Aylward 1969, 266–72).

As for the individual cases it reviewed, the Commission focused on ninety-nine cases where claims had been either rejected or never filed. It determined that, based on the criteria set out in its recommendations, fifty-two of these were entitled to compensation and forty-seven not entitled. Those judged to be not entitled were in two groups: cases not considered related to underground employment, including cardiovascular diseases, gastro-intestinal and urinary system diseases, and cancers other than lung and respiratory; and cases of individuals with no record of underground employment or with a record of underground employment "incompatible with disease causing disability or death" (Aylward 1969, 266–72). The Commission was careful to note that it did not have the final word on any case. Whether claims would ultimately be accepted or rejected depended on whether or not government accepted the relevant recommendations.

Notes

1. Lung Cancer – Progress Report, 18 November 1965, GN78/1/B, 220, File 290/G/07, PANL.
2. Report of a Visit to St. Lawrence, 18–22 September 1960, by Irving Fogwill, GN6, 3, PANL.
3. GN 6, 2, PANL.
4. Case Files, GN 6, 1, PANL.
5. Case Files, GN 6, 1, PANL.
6. Case Files, GN 6, 1, PANL.
7. L.G. Vey, Senior Administrative Assistant, Department of Health, Government of Newfoundland, to de Villiers, 16 February 1967, Health Survey — Burin Peninsula, GN 78/1/B, 220, File 290/G/01, PANL.
8. Vey to de Villiers, 17 February 1967, Health Survey — Burin Peninsula, GN 78/1/B, 220, File 290/G/01, PANL.
9. Press Release issued by Mr. R. Wiseman, General Manager, Newfoundland Fluorspar Limited, 17 February 1967, GN 6, 3, PANL.
10. Newfoundland Fluorspar Limited, Supplementary Submission to the Royal Commission on St. Lawrence: Rock-stress, Rock-bursts, Mining Methods, Newfluor Safety Policy and Practice, Accidents, Safety Training, GN 6, 3, PANL.

11. Leo Slaney to T. Alex Hickman, Minister of Justice, Government of Newfoundland, St. John's, 13 February 1967, MM.

12. Interview with Jerome Spearns, 28 November 1998.

13. Harry Ethridge, Public Relations Manager, Newfluor, to John C. Crosbie, Minister of Health, Government of Newfoundland, 10 May 1968, Survey Lung Cancer St. Lawrence Miners, GN 78/1/B, 220, File 290/G/07, PANL.

14. Report on the meeting held in St. John's 2 May 1968, to discuss the report of Professor Eric Trist, on the sociological aspects of the St. Lawrence problem, 2. MM.

15. T. Alex Hickman, Minister of Justice, Government of Newfoundland, to Leo Slaney, 6 April 1967, MM.

16. Newfoundland Fluorspar Limited, Submission to the Royal Commission on St. Lawrence, 33, GN 6, 3, PANL.

17. Newfoundland Fluorspar Limited, Submission to the Royal Commission on St. Lawrence, 27, GN 6, 3, PANL.

18. Newfoundland Fluorspar Limited, Submission to the Royal Commission on St. Lawrence, 176–77, GN 6, 3, PANL.

19. Transcript of a public hearing held at St. Lawrence, 27 November 1967, GN 6, 3, PANL, 25–27.

20. Transcript of a public hearing held at St. Lawrence, 27 November 1967, GN 6, 3, PANL, 73–80.

21. Fintan Aylward, Chairman, Royal Commission on St. Lawrence, Newfoundland, to S.T. Payne, CNTU, 9 October 1967, MM; and Aylward to Payne, 26 October 1967. MM.

22. Transcript of a public hearing held at St. Lawrence, 27 November 1967, GN 6, 3, PANL, 50–51.

23. Transcript of a public hearing held at St. Lawrence, 27 November 1967, GN 6, 3, PANL, 51–52.

24. Transcript of a public hearing held at St. Lawrence, 27 November 1967, GN 6, 3, PANL, 82, 107.

25. Transcript of a public hearing held at St. Lawrence, 27 November 1967, GN 6, 3, PANL, 122–23.

26. Transcript of a public hearing held at St. Lawrence, 27 November 1967, GN 6, 3, PANL, 47.

27. Transcript of a public hearing held at St. Lawrence, 27 November 1967, GN 6, 3, PANL, 210.

28. Transcript of a public hearing held at St. Lawrence, 27 November 1967, GN 6, 3, PANL, 215.

29. Fintan Aylward, Chairman, Royal Commission on St. Lawrence, to Robert Sauvé, General Secretary, CNTU, 19 December 1967, MM.

30. Leo Slaney to Marcel Pepin, President, CNTU, 4 December 1967, MM.

31. Leo Slaney to S.T. Payne, CNTU, 18 January 1968, MM.

32. St. Lawrence Workers Protective Union (CNTU), Submission to the Royal Commission on St. Lawrence, GN6, 3, PANL, 45.

33. St. Lawrence Workers Protective Union (CNTU), Submission to the Royal Commission on St. Lawrence, GN6, 3, PANL, 51.

34. St. Lawrence Workers Protective Union (CNTU), Submission to the Royal

Commission on St. Lawrence, GN6, 3, PANL, 90–91.
35. Town of St. Lawrence, Submission to the Royal Commission on St. Lawrence, GN 6, 3, PANL, 16.
36. Town of St. Lawrence, Submission to the Royal Commission on St. Lawrence, GN 6, 3, PANL, 6.
37. Town of St. Lawrence, Submission to the Royal Commission on St. Lawrence, GN 6, 3, PANL, 14.
38. St. Lawrence Workers Protective Union (CNTU), Submission to the Royal Commission on St. Lawrence, GN6, 3, PANL, 51.
39. Act No. 58, 1967. An Act to Amend the Workmen's Compensation Act, 1962. (A new consolidated Act was passed in 1962, embodying the amendments made since 1950.)
40. Case Files, GN 6, 1, PANL.
41. Case Files, GN 6, 1, PANL.

Chapter Six

MOUNTING PROTEST, INDUSTRY CLOSURE, AND THE LEGACY OF THE PAST

Reaction to the Royal Commission

While government and employers may have viewed the Royal Commission as a way of addressing the hostility and conflict that had come to pervade the St. Lawrence situation, the years immediately following the Commission's work would see the most turbulent and sustained labour unrest since the start of mining. The unrest would spread beyond the workplace and the labour relations realm into the community, drawing non-workers, most notably women, into the struggle to an unprecedented degree.

Much of the antagonism that marked the early 1970s grew out of the government's initial response to the Royal Commission's recommendations. The response, which came in May 1970, signalled movement on some areas, but this movement was limited, suggesting little tendency to break fundamentally with the status quo. For example, the government agreed to extend compensation coverage for loss of pulmonary function from uncertain causes, but only in cases where the worker had ceased employment after the Act came into effect in 1951. It also held to its refusal to recognize cases arising from lung cancer or silicosis before 1951. The only consideration given to pre-1951 claims was under the Special Fund that had been recommended by the Commission. Of the additional diseases the Commission had recommended for coverage — tuberculosis, any chronic obstructive pulmonary disease, and respiratory cancers other than lung cancer — the government agreed to include only silico-tuberculosis (Newfoundland 1970). This limited coverage benefitted only a small number of workers, those who had developed silico-tuberculosis and had terminated their employment after 1951. Ultimately, the response meant that of the fifty-two claims the Royal Commission had recommended for approval under its criteria, only seven would be accepted.

In response to the recommendation that a second government radiation monitor be employed at St. Lawrence, the government proposed that in the future radiation monitoring would be the responsibility of the company (Newfoundland 1970). This proposal grew out of a suggestion made several months earlier by Mines Minister W.R. Callahan, who hoped that Newfluor would employ the government monitor then in St. Lawrence and thus free up resources to allow the Mines Inspection Division to hire a clerk.[1]

Not surprisingly, the government's response to the Royal Commission's recommendations drew sharp criticism from some quarters. The union described it as another demonstration of the government's lack of regard for the "misery and suffering that have faced the widows and dependents of deceased and disabled miners."[2] The union also charged that the plan to withdraw the government radiation monitor threatened what little progress had been made in that area in recent years, and revealed that the government's real agenda in appointing the monitor in 1967 was "to bury a very controversial issue that was a source of embarrassment to the Government."[3]

The response also became a subject of controversy in the political arena. The district's member in the provincial legislature (who had recently defected from Smallwood's Liberals to the Progressive Conservatives) charged that by handing responsibility for radiation monitoring over to the company the government was abdicating its duty to protect the health of St. Lawrence miners (*Evening Telegram* June 3, 1970). Called on repeatedly to defend this decision, the Mines Minister simply stated that the company had a "legal and moral responsibility" to protect the health of its employees. Reminded of the union's warning that this decision would increase suspicion and unrest at St. Lawrence, Callahan only repeated that the law required operators to ensure that their mines were safe (Newfoundland 1970b, 6137–45).

The government also came under fire for its response to the matter of workers' compensation, particularly with respect to widows' benefits. Criticism over this issue was intensified by the results of a survey conducted by the provincial Department of Health and Welfare just prior to release of the government's response to the Royal Commission. The survey, carried out at the request of the union, looked into the circumstances of about twenty widows in St. Lawrence and confirmed what many already knew — that compensation benefits were inadequate and families were living in sub-standard housing. However, it concluded that little could be done except to advise these women of their right to apply for welfare to supplement their compensation benefits. Many widows apparently refused to apply for welfare on the grounds that they and their children were entitled to a sufficient income from workers' compensation (Newfoundland 1970b, 6431–33). The report also suggested that widows try to supplement their incomes through such activities as "small scale gardening, berry picking, mending and sewing."[4]

Criticism of the government's response to the recommendations continued through 1970. In November the Commission Chair himself wrote to the Premier charging that the government had essentially ignored the recommendations regarding compensation.[5]

"We Support our Husbands": The First Women's Protest and the 1971 Strike

Alongside these ongoing complaints over the response to the Royal Commission, relations between the company and its workers apparently continued to deteriorate. Vandalism and theft of company property increased to the point where the company hired professional security guards (*Newfluor News* June, 1969, 3). At the same time, Newfluor continued its efforts to create a positive image and to build good will, sponsoring community events and organizations, and using the *Newfluor News* to combat fears about health and safety and to congratulate workers on maintaining high production levels.

The company's efforts at building better labour relations were no doubt motivated by its desire to continue expanding operations and increasing production. By 1970 the Tarefare mine had also been put back into production for the first time since the Second World War, milling and loading facilities were being upgraded and expanded, and Newfluor employed about 350 workers. The company shipped a record amount of fluorspar in 1970, an increase of about 40 percent over the previous year. Plans were also underway to open a third mine at the old Blue Beach site, which Alcan had purchased from the St. Lawrence Corporation in 1965 (Canada, Department of Mines and Technical Surveys 1970, 227–28).

The union sought to share in the company's apparent prosperity when it entered negotiations for renewal of its collective agreement in 1971, requesting an across-the-board increase of $1.25 per hour, which would have given St. Lawrence workers wage parity with those at the Arvida smelter.[6] The union's prediction of "hard bargaining ahead" turned out to be accurate.[7] After three months of negotiations and a failed attempt at government conciliation, talks broke down (*Evening Telegram* April 7, 1971, 3).

On April 6, shortly after the breakdown in talks, matters took an unusual turn when about thirty women from St. Lawrence and nearby Lawn started picketing the loading dock to prevent an ore carrier from loading a shipment for Arvida. After spending the night at the dock under observation by several RCMP officers, they were joined the next day by about ten other women. The union was reportedly not officially backing this protest, but workers made no effort to cross the line and load the vessel (*Evening Telegram* April 6, 1971, 3). The women stayed on the dock for two days and nights, many carrying placards reading "We Support Our Husbands." Esther Spracklin, spokeswoman for the group, stated that they believed that allowing the ore to be loaded would undercut the union's bargaining position. The protest ended on April 8 when the carrier sailed without having loaded the ore (*Evening Telegram* April 8, 1971, 3).

Though brief, the women's protest was significant in a number of respects. On one level, it was a response to their immediate circumstances. Women had long suffered the effects of industrial disease — caring for dying husbands or fathers, raising children with little financial support, and living with the constant fear that their husband or son might be next. In fact, Esther Spracklin's father had died of industrial disease and her husband was a miner. Though the women had tried through various channels to draw attention to their plight in the past, the 1971 protest was their first concerted, public action.

On another level, the women's protests can be viewed in the context of the general climate of unrest and protest within the province at the time. In the political arena Smallwood's Liberal government was losing the grip it had held since 1949. The government was being undermined and challenged from many quarters, including the media, the arts community, and a group of highly vocal Progressive Conservative politicians (Gillespie 1986, 130–32). In a place where one leader and one party had held such dominance for so long, this attack was about more than political change — it was a manifestation of social unrest and a growing culture of protest. At the same time, a wave of labour unrest was sweeping the province. About a week before St. Lawrence miners took to the picket line, members of the United Steelworkers of America union at a copper mine in Springdale, on the northeast coast, had gone on strike to demand increased wages and improved benefits (*Evening Telegram* April 12, 1971). Shortly thereafter, the Newfoundland Fishermen, Food and Allied Workers' Union began what would become a long series of strikes and protests around the island, bringing to over 1,000 the number of workers from various sectors on strike around the province (*Evening Telegram* April 19, 1971). By the end of 1971, there would be twenty-nine strikes involving nearly 6,000 workers, compared to eight involving fewer than 1,000 workers the previous year (Kealey 1986, 112).

The women's actions can also be viewed against the background of another general development taking place at the time, as women across Canada and elsewhere were challenging and breaking out of their traditional roles and taking a more active role in politics, the labour movement, and other public venues. While there is no direct evidence of a connection between this broader trend and events at St. Lawrence, it is nonetheless difficult to imagine women there taking such action even five years earlier.

After overwhelmingly rejecting the company's most recent wage offer, on April 18, 1971, the workers went on strike (*Evening Telegram* April 16, 1971; April 18, 1971). The specific matter at stake was wages; however, the strike was played out against the backdrop of ongoing grievances over other issues. The government was drawing criticism for inaction on establishing the Special Fund, which it had promised to do more than a year earlier with the assistance of employers (*Evening Telegram* April 2, 1971). It had also been revealed that in 1970 Alcan had entered into an agreement to purchase fluorspar from a Mexican supplier and that shipments of that ore were to commence shortly.

The knowledge that Alcan was turning to Mexican suppliers naturally did not sit well with workers at St. Lawrence, given their experience with the St. Lawrence Corporation (*Evening Telegram* April 10, 1970). The unions directly linked wages to health and safety hazards, arguing that its requested wage hike would not only help keep pace with the rising cost of living but also help compensate for the special dangers encountered by St. Lawrence miners. CNTU representative Peter Curtis noted that that the company would have a more difficult time bargaining than it had in the past, as it was now dealing with a "new breed of worker" in St. Lawrence, "men who had watched their fathers and relations snuffed out in the prime of life by lung cancer or mine accidents, men who have seen these same fathers and relations taken advantage of in other wage settlements" (*Evening Telegram* May 7, 1971).

As an indication of the growing solidarity between the workforce and the community, in May a group of women took over the picket lines while striking miners marched a coffin and a cancer symbol through the town to the cemetery (*Evening Telegram* May 10, 1971). The government's response to this event, widely covered in the media, marked the beginning of a pattern that would be repeated several times during the 1970s: granting concessions on workplace health and workers' compensation issues in an attempt to quell unrest. Shortly after the protest march, the government changed its earlier position and proposed that the government radiation monitor be posted permanently in St. Lawrence at government expense (*Evening Telegram* May 14, 1971). A month later, the government introduced changes to the Workmen's Compensation Act that reflected some of its decisions on the recommendations of the Royal Commission. Monthly payments for widows and dependents were increased, and the monthly ceiling on widows' benefits was eliminated (Newfoundland 1972).

Various parties, including the union and the St. Lawrence Town Council, also continued to press the government on the matter of establishing the Special Fund. The provincial government claimed that it and Alcan had agreed to contribute, but there had been no response from either the federal government or anyone associated with the St. Lawrence Corporation.[8] By July 1971, the provincial government and Alcan had apparently given up hope that the federal government or the St. Lawrence Corporation would contribute to the fund and decided to proceed without them. No doubt motivated by a desire to end the ongoing labour dispute and get back into production, Alcan urged the provincial government to make an announcement to that effect "as quickly as possible."[9]

The labour dispute also served to draw attention to other issues in the community, including perceived social problems. It was reported that a higher than average number of young people in St. Lawrence were drug users. The parish priest, RCMP, and town residents attributed this to a number of

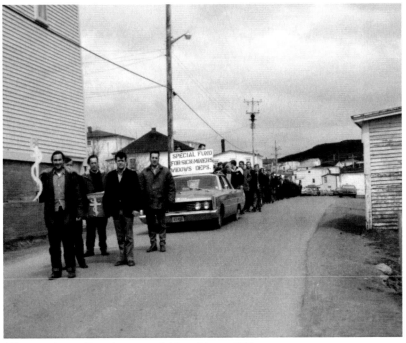

Miners carrying a coffin and cancer symbol through town, 1971.

factors. It was suggested that as an industrial community, St. Lawrence was not like other, more traditional Newfoundland communities and that people there were more apt to "try new things," including drugs. Others pointed out that there were no recreational facilities in the community, though Newfluor had for years been promising to help fund construction of such a facility. The most common reasons offered for the reportedly high rate of drug use, however, were that many households lacked a father figure to instill a strong sense of discipline in their children, and that the high death rate in the community had instilled in young people the attitude that they should "eat, drink, and be merry for tomorrow we may die" (*Evening Telegram* June 30, 1975, 1). In the absence of any hard evidence about the rate of drug use at St. Lawrence compared to other communities, it is difficult to say whether these claims were accurate. Nonetheless, they were significant in that they illustrate growing interest in the social and psychological effects of industrial disease on families and households in the community.

The media continued to publicize the plight of widows. A newspaper report in early July described how one woman whose husband was classed as 80 percent disabled and unable to earn any other income struggled to raise six children on $158 a month. Others talked of having no social life because they could not afford even the small amount of money needed to attend community events (*Evening Telegram* July 6, 1971, 1). Negative publicity of this kind continued throughout the summer of 1971. A dying miner interviewed in the St. Lawrence hospital talked of regretting "every day I worked in the mine" and of his frustration in trying to get financial support for his family (*Evening Telegram* July 8, 1971).

Given this type of publicity and the fact that the provincial government was barely clinging to power with an election imminent, it is understandable that some took a cynical view of a July 1971 announcement that government representatives, including Smallwood, would go to St. Lawrence soon to announce the establishment of the Special Fund. Satirist Ray Guy, a constant thorn in Smallwood's side, noted that after years of neglect and procrastination and with an election two months away, the "Smallwood flying circus" was off to St. Lawrence to "wring from the sorrow and torment of widows and orphans a few more filthy votes" (*Evening Telegram* July 6, 1971).

Underlying tensions continued to flare up as the dispute dragged on. Striking workers became more resentful of non-unionized staff members who were doing maintenance jobs such as keeping the mine pumps running. Workers also complained that the company was fuelling anger by delivering hampers of food and bottles of wine to these staff members' houses and continuing to host weekly parties at the Staff House. Both the union president and the town's long-time resident physician, Dr. Brian Hollywood, charged that the company was manipulating media coverage and using channels like the *Newfluor News* to present a distorted version of the situation. The union president claimed that many things he had reported or submitted to the *Newfluor News* had been altered without his knowledge or consent before publication. The company denied all such allegations (*Evening Telegram* July 9, 1971).

It was in this climate of tension and distrust that in August Smallwood made his promised trip to St. Lawrence and announced the establishment of the Special Fund to be jointly financed by Alcan and the provincial government. Even this became a target of criticism. Former Royal Commission Chair Fintan Aylward remarked that while the establishment of the Special Fund would undoubtedly benefit some families, more effort should have been made to locate parties associated with the St. Lawrence Corporation and to force them to contribute (*Evening Telegram* August 2, 1971). Another commentator welcomed the financial help, but rued the fact that people had been forced to wait for it while the Smallwood government improved its Liberal candidate's election chances (*Evening Telegram* August 2, 1971).

The provincial government and Alcan originally contributed $500,000 each to the fund, to be paid out at a rate of $100,000 per year. Fifty-one claimants already in receipt of workers' compensation began receiving Special Fund payments. It was anticipated that at least thirty others would eventually qualify for the Special Fund, while seventy other cases were under medical review by the WCB. The monthly payments turned out to be abysmally low. The head of a family — a disabled miner or widow — would receive $30.86 a month, the wife of a disabled miner $15.43 a month, and dependent children just $7.72 per month. The highest amount paid out in the initial qualifying group was $100.34, to a family consisting of two parents and seven dependent children.[10]

Newfluor was quick to point out that it had proposed the Special Fund in its brief to the Royal Commission and that Alcan had shown not only a willingness to contribute to the fund but "an anxiety to see it established" (*Newfluor News* September 1971). This is understandable, given what the Special Fund meant in terms of financial liability. The taxpayers of the province directly contributed half of the money required for the fund, allowing the company to evade its financial responsibility for the disaster once again, just as it had done about a decade earlier when cancer claims were charged to the WCB's Disaster Fund. The St. Lawrence Corporation, meanwhile, paid nothing into the Special Fund and thus continued to shirk all responsibility for its role in the disaster.

Shortly after the announcement of the Special Fund, the union and the company reached an agreement to settle the strike. Union president Leo Slaney noted that while the wage increase under the agreement was considerably less than the amount initially sought, gains had been made in other areas, including seniority, sick benefits, and annual vacations. He also pointed out that the strike had been instrumental in getting the company and the government to establish the Special Fund. However, it was clear that the deal did not have solid support among the membership, winning only 60 percent support for ratification (*Evening Telegram* September 11, 1971). Shortly thereafter, the union president resigned and took a non-union position with the company, whereupon vice-president George Doyle became the acting president (*Evening Telegram* September 30, 1971).

Buying Peace: Agitation and Change, 1973–74

Early in 1972, the company finally gave in to persistent demands from the union to hire a second radiation monitor. The Newfluor manager told the Department of Mines that he believed this was of little practical benefit, since the company's monitoring and reduction program was sufficient; however, he also conceded that hiring the government's monitor, David Rex, might help build trust, since "the miners trust Mr. Rex's results more than they do our monitors, even though the actual data collected are similar."[11] Under the new system, areas which regularly gave no cause for concern would be tested weekly, those which usually gave readings up to 0.1 times the SWL twice weekly, and those with readings in excess of 0.1 times the SWL daily.

The company suggested that these tests be cross-checked by the government monitor as often as deemed appropriate. Despite the company's stated confidence in its ability to control radiation levels, readings in excess of the SWL continued to be recorded. At least fourteen such readings were obtained by the company monitors from March to September 1972, and in September the government monitor reported a reading of twenty-eight times the SWL at Director mine.[12]

A change of government in 1972 brought further amendments to workers' compensation coverage. In March of that year, the Smallwood Liberals were finally ousted, replaced by the Progressive Conservatives under Frank Moores. Having spent much of the previous few years hammering the Liberals over their response to the St. Lawrence situation, the new government likely felt compelled to take some action. Soon after taking office, it amended the Act to cover two further groups of claimants. The first was workers employed underground at a St. Lawrence mine between 1951 and 1960 whose disablement or death had been caused by any chronic obstructive pulmonary disease. This amendment in coverage recognized that although a causal connection between working conditions and certain pulmonary diseases could not be conclusively established in some cases, "rational observation indicates the probability of such a connection." The second group was those listed in the Report of the Royal Commission as being entitled to compensation under the recommendations. Compensation for such cases would continue to be drawn from the Disaster Fund (Newfoundland 1973).

While these amendments represented important gains, the union continued to press for expanded coverage. In November 1972, it urged the government to extend coverage to those who had worked in surface areas such as the processing mill and crushing plant and had developed pulmonary diseases but were not covered because they had not worked as "miners" or underground. The union rejected the implication in the 1972 amendment that the health hazard from radiation and dust ceased to exist after 1960. It also continued to demand that coverage be extended to all those who had become disabled prior to 1951, pointing to the absurdity in compensating some such claimants simply because they had been listed in the Royal Commission report, and refusing to consider other potential claims arising before that date simply because they were not listed.[13]

The union also continued to complain to the government about the fact that benefits were based on wages at the time of disablement. To stress the psychological as well as the financial burden this entailed, the union pointed out "a tragic fact": because the calculation of death benefits was based upon a set amount, regardless of earnings, "some such men live in the realization that rather than [contributing] to their dependents' welfare they are an obvious burden, in that compensation payable will increase on their deaths."[14]

Once again, action on these demands came only in the context of further labour unrest. As an indication that the labour relations environment continued to be antagonistic, less than twenty-four hours after the collective agreement expired the union voted 90 percent in favour of a strike and set up picket lines (*Evening Telegram* April 2, 1973). St. Lawrence workers were again part of a wave of labour unrest across the province. When the SLWPU went out on April 1, it joined 600 other workers from the construction, petroleum refining, and fish processing industries already on strike, plus nearly 600 miners on strike at the Buchans mine (*Evening Telegram* April 7, 1973).

A month into the strike, the government passed yet more amendments to the Workmen's Compensation Act (*Evening Telegram* May 2, 1973). These changes again increased monthly payment to widows and dependent children, and they extended coverage for lung cancer and silicosis to workers employed underground at St. Lawrence, before or after 1951. They also allowed claims arising from work in "fluorspar extraction or handling, or both, at St. Lawrence," thus covering workers not employed underground at the time of their disability (Newfoundland 1974). Just two days after these amendments were made, the union membership voted in favour of an offer giving them wage increases and requiring the transfer and retraining of workers who could no longer work underground for health reasons (*Evening Telegram* May 4, 1973).

Taking advantage of a relatively peaceful period on the labour relations front, Newfluor increased production in 1974 and began work on a second shaft at the Tarefare mine. That new shaft was scheduled to go into production in 1976 (*Newfluor News* 1974). However, while there were no open labour disputes, the union persisted with complaints about inadequate ventilation and about the high radiation levels being detected by both company and government monitors at the Director, Tarefare, and Blue Beach mines.[15]

The company, meanwhile, continued to use various, sometimes questionable means to polish its corporate image. For instance, a *Newfluor News* article quoted the praise of Mayor Jules Mirault for the company's community improvement efforts. In addition to being mayor, Mirault had been hired in 1972 as the company's radiation technician (*Newfluor News* June, 1974). Some of the company's public relations efforts appear absurd under the circumstances. The December 1974 issue of the *Newfluor News*, for example, carried an advertisement for a book on making Christmas crafts and decorations using Alcan aluminum foil, available to Newfluor employees for the "special low price" of $3 (*Newfluor News* December, 1974).

"An Emotional Feeling of Bitterness": Labour and Community Unrest, 1975–76

While 1974 had been a relatively calm year, 1975 would be an entirely different matter. With the collective agreement coming up for renewal, Alcan began early in that year to describe its alleged financial woes. The February issue of the *Newfluor News* carried an extensive article on the impact of a recessionary downturn on Alcan and predictions for a "tough year ahead" (*Newfluor News* February, 1975). In fact, production had declined by about 15 percent from 1974 to 1975, leaving Alcan's Quebec smelters operating at slightly reduced capacity (Litvak and Maule 1977, 91, 150). Technological changes in the smelting process had also reduced the amount of fluorspar required per ton of raw aluminum. The company nonetheless continued to show substantial profits, $169 million (U.S.) in 1974 and $35 million (U.S.) in 1975 (Litvak and Maule 1977, 206).

Apparently unmoved by Alcan's claims about its economic woes, the CNTU urged the SLWPU to press hard for a wage increase to keep pace with the rising cost of living and to address the inequity in wages among Alcan employees across the country. The CNTU pointed out that a recent settlement had given workers at Alcan's smelter in Kitimat, British Columbia, about $2.30 more per hour than workers in St. Lawrence, despite the fact that the cost of living was higher in Newfoundland than in British Columbia and that any recent increases received by Newfoundland and Quebec workers had been erased by inflation. The CNTU described this as an instance of regional disparity and oppression, claiming that Alcan had divided its Canadian workers into three classes: "A top-rated class of workers out west, a second class in Quebec, and a third class in Newfoundland."[16]

The CNTU's language and its position, along with much of what ultimately transpired at St. Lawrence, must be viewed in the context of the environment in Quebec and the organization's overall agenda. As with many parts of Canada, Quebec in the early 1970s was subject to high inflation and unemployment, which contributed to a wave of labour and public unrest. What distinguished the situation in Quebec was a growing tendency to relate these economic issues to political factors, giving rise to a marriage of the labour movement and the separatist movement. Within this environment, the CNTU deepened its commitment to Quebec independence and to political radicalism. For instance, in 1971 the CNTU began issuing attacks on the capitalist system itself, identifying it with imperialist domination of Quebec by Anglo-Canadian and American interests (including Alcan) and calling on the Quebec labour movement to devote itself to "Québécois socialism" (CNTU 248–49; Desrosiers and Héroux 1973, 155–56; Güntzel 2000).

Not everyone agreed with the CNTU's move in a more radical direction: during 1972 the organization lost about 70,000 members, about one-third of its membership. About half of these joined a breakaway organization known as the Confederation des Syndicats Democratique (CSD) (Rouillard 1981, 233–38). Among the unions to break with the CNTU were many of those in the Metal Trades Federation, including those in the Quebec aluminum sector. By the end of 1973, about 9,000 such workers, or one-third of the Metal Trades Federation membership, had left the CNTU to join the CSD or another parent body, or to become independent. The Arvida union joined the independent Fédération des syndicats du secteur de l'aluminum (FSSA) (Rouillard 1981, 238, 260).

Following the shift to a more radical program during the early 1970s, the CNTU and many other Quebec labour organizations engaged in a series of militant job actions. Members of a Quebec Federation of Labour (QFL) union held out for nine months during 1973–74 at the American-owned Firestone tire plant in Joliette and walked out again in a wildcat strike in the summer of 1974. CNTU-affiliated workers at Canadian Gypsum walked off the job in May 1973 and won their demands after a twenty-month strike. In August 1973, 400 workers from twenty companies occupied the offices of the Quebec Department of Labour to demand anti-scab legislation. In January 1974, 2,000 members of the United Aeronautics Workers (of the QFL) at the Longueuil aircraft plant walked off in what became one of the longest and most bitter strikes in Canadian history, lasting until the summer of 1975. Workers at the Montreal Transit Commission staged a victorious forty-four-day strike over cost-of-living increases in the summer of 1974, and in October of that year 40,000 construction workers staged a demonstration in Montreal over the issue of wage indexation (CNTU 241–46; Rouillard 1981, 177–210). It is not surprising, therefore, that on the advice of the CNTU the SLWPU's 1975 demands included a substantial wage increase, a cost-of-living allowance, and other improvements, along with more frequent radiation monitoring and increased union representation on the Safety Committee.

In early June, the women of the community once again became publicly engaged in the union's struggle, but this time on a much larger scale. Shortly after the company presented what it claimed was its final wage offer, a group of about 200 women again occupied the wharf and blocked the ore carrier from taking on a load of fluorspar (*Evening Telegram* June 27, 1975). Twelve days into the blockade, after its request for an injunction to have the women removed was denied, the company suspended all operations.[17]

The union claimed workers were locked out, but the company insisted they were laid off because of the halt in production caused by the "unreasonable and unauthorized actions of the women" (*Evening Telegram* June 11, 1975). Esther Spracklin, who was once again the spokeswoman for the group, stated that their actions had simply delayed the lockout and given the men some paid work they would not have otherwise had. Furthermore, she said, the union would have prevented the boat from loading anyway, and the women had prevented workers from having to resort to strike action, which they wanted to avoid if possible (*Evening Telegram* June 11, 1975).

The 1975 blockade generated strong and diverse responses. The union

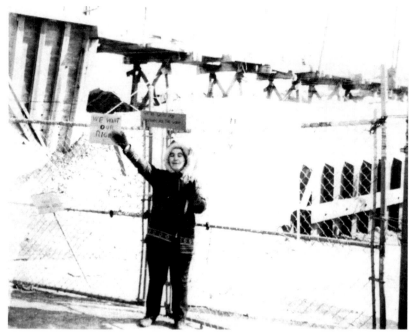

Protestor at the loading dock, 1975. The sign over her right hand says, "We want our rights," and the one above her head says, "We're with our miners all the way."

claimed it did not officially support the blockade, yet workers refused to cross the women's line to load the ore carrier (*Evening Telegram* June 11, 1975). One worker later stated, "We thought they were doing the right thing; we wanted to stop the ore from going."[18] As a local man in middle management recalled, when Newfluor management heard the day before the blockade a rumour that the women would engage in this action, they became deeply concerned over the potential effects. They believed the dispute would take a "very different turn" once women became involved in this way, and they were also troubled by how their actions might draw further media and public attention to the dispute and more widespread sympathy for the workers and their cause.[19] Management's agitation over the blockade was apparent in its demand to a group of workers that they "go out and get that mess cleaned up" (*Evening Telegram* June 11, 1975).

As an indication of the level of tension, the day after the company shut down the mines about fifty workers, in a move reportedly not sanctioned by the union, occupied the pay office and demanded the company issue lay-off slips so that they could apply for Unemployment Insurance (UI) benefits. Otherwise, the men would receive only strike pay ($30 per week for single men and $50 per week for married men.) Six of the men were arrested and charged with "intimidating by violence" and participating in an "unlawful assembly." Miners used the court appearance in mid-June as a display of solidarity: a large group of miners accompanied the accused men on the fifty-kilometre trip to the courthouse (*Evening Telegram* June 12, 1975).

CNTU representative Peter Curtis, who was at this event, insisted that if authorities were looking for evidence of violence they should look to the cemetery, where there was "a whole graveyard of blood and violence." Curtis also pointed out that the labour dispute was about more than wages: it was also about the history of death and disease in St. Lawrence and the inadequacy of financial support for widows and disabled miners (*Evening Telegram* June 12, 1975). Given that five miners, all under fifty years old, had died during late 1974 and early 1975 (*Evening Telegram* June 21, 1975), Curtis's comments no doubt had a particular resonance.

The mounting death toll also likely influenced the actions of the women who continued to support the union and the workers publicly. As spokeswoman Spracklin pointed out, she and many of these women not only had husbands working in the mines, many of them had watched their fathers and other relatives die and were determined not to repeat that history. Spracklin stated that the women were directly affected by what happened to their husbands, in terms of both wages and working conditions. "What happens to the men," she said, "affects all of us. Any one of us could join the nearly 200 widows in the community, and I say we're involved!" (*Evening Telegram* June 29, 1975).

The fiery rhetoric of the CNTU and the women protesters was paralleled by the increasingly aggressive actions of the workers. The same day as the court appearance for the six accused men (which resulted in a postponement of the case), over a hundred miners went to the Newfluor payroll office demanding lay-off slips. They were met by five RCMP officers. The men threatened that there would be trouble if their layoff slips stated "labour dispute" as this would deny them UI benefits. When the men were told they would be permitted into the office only one at a time, they began pushing up against the door and hurling insults at the police. When the first worker emerged from the building and informed the others that the slips said "labour dispute," the enraged men vowed not to let company staff tending the mine pumps enter the mine at the four o'clock shift change or let personnel leave the pay office at five o'clock. The RCMP summoned fourteen officers from neigbouring towns to stand by in the community, dressed in riot gear. A full-blown confrontation was averted when the union executive informed the men that negotiations had resumed and called them to a meeting at the union hall, where they were ordered not to return to the pay office that night (*Evening Telegram* June 13, 1975).

As the dispute dragged on through the summer of 1975, it became a flashpoint for many long-festering grievances. Bud Loder stated that the dispute was about a host of issues, including "wages, and safety and ventila-tion." "Ventilation was better than in earlier years," he said, "but we still got high readings."[20] Peter Curtis reiterated this position, pointing out that while wages were the most prominent issue at stake, the union was also concerned about health and safety and workers' compensation (*Evening Telegram* June 14, 1975.) The Newfluor manager himself noted that antagonism over these issues continued to pervade the company's relations with the workers and the community. "There's an emotional feeling of bitterness against Alcan," he said, "which exists all the time below the surface. A lot of it is ancient history, dating back to pre-Alcan years, but this feeling comes up every time we come to negotiations" (*Evening Telegram* June 14, 1975).

The continuing agitation for further improvements to workers' compen-sation coverage paid off yet again in June 1975, with the passage of another amendment to the Act. The amendments of 1972 and 1973 had been based on the assumption that there was no risk of those diseases among workers who began work after 1960, an assumption the union had vigorously opposed. The 1975 amendment extended coverage to silicosis and cancer contracted after 1960 (Newfoundland 1976).

The CNTU's rhetoric was clearly influencing the thinking of some rank and file members. One young worker — among the group that Curtis had called the "new breed" of Newfluor employee — used the very language of the CNTU when he claimed that Alcan viewed St. Lawrence workers as "third-class citizens" within its hierarchy of Canadian workers. Management, meanwhile, detected and resented this influence, claiming that much of the problem with labour relations in St. Lawrence arose from the fact that the local union was being "led astray by an outside union" (*Evening Telegram* June 21, 1975).

Events in 1975 also underscored the social stratification that had emerged in the community, especially between workers and management. One worker claimed that management did not associate with workers because they felt they were "too good for the likes of us." As an example, he pointed out that Alcan had built a curling rink at the Staff Club near the management homes, but neither he nor his fellow workers "would think of going up there" (*Evening Telegram* June 21, 1975). One former worker recalled that there was far more of this social differentiation in St. Lawrence, where one's social position was determined by one's job, than in other Newfoundland communities.[21] The 1975 dispute put some locals who were members of management into an uncomfortable position. "We were staff," one such person recalled, "but we also knew what the people had suffered and continued to suffer. We had a lot of compassion but our issue was how do we salvage the industry? Where does your allegiance lie? You're torn."[22]

In September, Newfluor tried to pressure workers into accepting its wage offer by telling them that the company had already purchased half its winter supply of fluorspar from Mexico and was prepared to purchase the remainder there if need be. If that purchase went ahead, management stated, no ore would be shipped from St. Lawrence until at least the following year. However, the union simply professed confusion at the company's position and the implied ultimatum, questioning why the company persisted in treating the matter as a labour dispute when in fact it was a lay-off, one that allowed the company to get cheaper fluorspar in Mexico and that had been falsely justified on the grounds that the women had blocked the ore boat from loading (*Evening Telegram* October 22, 1975).

According to the union president, morale remained high and the men were determined not to return to work under the company's conditions, though they conceded that they were facing a tough winter if they did not qualify for UI and had to live on strike pay (*Evening Telegram* September 29, 1975). In mid-November word came that the workers would not qualify for UI, since they had been laid off because of a labour dispute (*Evening Telegram* November 10, 1975, November 14, 1975).

While the company attempted to make wages the sole issue at stake, the union continued to force the issue of health and safety. Only three days after the UI ruling, SLWPU and CNTU representatives met with government officials to recommend specific changes to the Mine Safety Regulations, including frequent tests of pulmonary function in miners and personal monitoring devices to assess individual radiation exposure. The miners were assured that new regulations would be on the books early in the following year (*Evening Telegram* November 14, 1975). The CNTU also called on the provincial government to institute measures guaranteeing workers' rights to know about potential health risks in the workplace and to refuse unsafe work.[23] Eventually the "Right to Know" and the "Right to Refuse" would become standard features of health and safety law across Canada, though they were cutting-edge notions at the time the CNTU was pressing for them.

Another element of the broader context in which events at St. Lawrence unfolded in the mid-1970s was a growing awareness of the human health and environmental effects of such industries as copper, asbestos, and uranium mining, as well as heightened worker and public concern about such issues in Canada, the United States, and elsewhere (Ashford 1976, 3–4; Reschenthaler 1979, 13). One commentator noted in the late 1970s: "There has been rarely a week in the past two or three years when some major Canadian newspaper did not contain at least one story related to occupational health" (Paehlke 1979, 97–98).

This increased awareness and concern was evident in the fact that elsewhere across the country the effects of various health hazards in mining were being investigated and exposed. For example, in Ontario, a Royal

Commission on the Health and Safety of Workers in Mines (the "Ham Commission") was exploring how years of neglect, jurisdictional confusion, and bureaucratic wrangling had led to deaths and disease among miners at Elliot Lake uranium mines (Ham 1975, 79–80). In Quebec, the Comité d' étude sur la salubrité dans l' industrie de l'aminante was studying the health effects of asbestos mining and milling. In fact, during 1975 the CNTU was deeply involved in a struggle over the asbestos issue in Quebec: that year 3,000 CNTU- affiliated workers staged a seven-month strike at the Thetford mines, eventually forcing the Quebec government to pass more stringent dust control regulations and to compensate victims of asbestosis and silicosis (Rouillard 1981, 261). Within the province of Newfoundland, health and safety was also becoming a key concern among iron ore miners in Labrador and asbestos miners at Baie Verte (Newfoundland 1979; Labrador Institute of Northern Studies 1982; Martland 1978).

Public and media attention continued to play an important role in the St. Lawrence situation. An important development in this respect was the publication of Elliot Leyton's *Dying Hard* (1975a), containing a series of interviews he had conducted with ailing miners and with women in the community. Through its revelations about the physical, emotional, and psychological pain inflicted by industrial disease and the frustrating and often humiliating ordeal of seeking workers' compensation benefits, the book drew a great deal of public and media attention to the St. Lawrence disaster. Leyton appeared on national radio and television programs as part of a national publicity tour (Leyton 1977a). Because the book was designed as social advocacy rather than an academic study, it also garnered a lot of coverage in the popular press (Leyton 1975b). A Newfoundland theatre troupe, "The Mummers," which used theatre as a vehicle for social advocacy, toured a play called "Dying Hard," and the CBC produced an hour-long feature based on the book (Leyton 1977a). Leyton also used his work in St. Lawrence as the basis for a submission to the government and the WCB critiquing their response to the St. Lawrence disaster and making a number of recommendations (Leyton 1977a), which were, apparently, completely ignored (Leyton 1977b).

In December 1975 actors and musicians staged a benefit concert for the miners in St. John's, an event that raised over $6,000. CNTU representative Michel Chartrand used the occasion not only to reiterate the organization's commitment to the St. Lawrence miners, but also as a forum for airing the CNTU's more general aims and grievances. This included a wholesale denunciation of capitalists as "sophisticated legal crooks" and a blistering attack on the federal government of Pierre Trudeau and the wage and price controls it had introduced two months earlier, despite having opposed the suggestion in the election campaign of 1974 (*Evening Telegram* December 12, 1975). Like many other Canadian labour organizations, the CNTU denounced the requirement under the wage control policy that proposed wage increases be submitted to the Anti-Inflation Board for approval; the CNTU viewed this requirement as an attack on workers' rights and on the collective bargaining system (CNTU 222–41).

While the CNTU continued to pledge its allegiance to St. Lawrence workers holding out against the company, the SLWPU was being subjected to increasing pressure to settle. Shortly before Christmas, with the strike in its ninth month, the company offered members a lump sum of $500 each to accept its latest wage offer. The membership rejected the proposal,[24] and its rejection was quickly followed by a letter reminding workers that while Alcan would keep its St. Lawrence mines open if it could be assured an "uninterrupted supply," it had the option of obtaining fluorspar cheaper in Mexico.[25] The mayor, who was also a member of Newfluor staff, expressed dismay that the union had rejected the most recent offer, and he suggested that the men would have accepted the offer had they not been under the sway of Curtis and the CNTU. He agreed with the company — his employer — that the actions of the union were threatening the future of the St. Lawrence mines (*Evening Telegram* December 20, 1975).

At the end of January 1976, the company turned up the pressure again by announcing that it was shutting down the mines for an "indefinite period." Newfluor claimed it was disappointed this action had to be taken but defended itself by arguing that the union had stubbornly refused its best offer despite the fact that cheaper fluorspar could be had elsewhere (*Evening Telegram* February 2, 1976). The provincial government announced that it was preparing back-to-work legislation to force the miners back. In the context of these threats, the parties went back to the table and soon reached an agreement. In addition to wage increases, the agreement called for the training of a radiation monitor from within the union membership.[26] It was approved by 75 percent of voting members (*Evening Telegram* February 7, 1976).

Union president Michael Slaney explained that the union had been forced to choose "the lesser of two evils… to stay off the job and have legislation forced upon us [or] to accept this contract proposal." He also noted that the constant threat of having the mines closed permanently was a risk the union just "couldn't afford" to take. On the positive side, he said, the union had made the company move slightly on the wage issue and the strike had been about more than wages; it had also been about "integrity and principle." Asked whether he thought the strike had damaged relations between the company and the union, Slaney said no, "we've never had a normal relationship with them anyway" (*Evening Telegram* February 7, 1976).

Industry Closure, 1976–1978

Just as the industry was getting back on track following the strike, developments elsewhere began to have an adverse effect on the St. Lawrence operation. In June 1976, about 8,000 workers at three of Alcan's Quebec plants (members of the FSSA unions that had broken away from the CNTU a few years earlier) went on strike to demand wage increases.[27] The strike shut down the Arvida plant, and by July Newfluor had laid off about half of the 250 workers re-hired to that point (*Evening Telegram* July 12, 1976). The Arvida strike finally ended in November 1976, but reactivation of the plant took considerable time. Total fluorspar shipments for 1976 were about half the normal amount, and at the end of that year there were just over a hundred workers on the job.[28]

The new year brought little cause for optimism. In February 1977, Newfluor informed the union that while it planned to increase production and put the mines on two shifts, it was concerned about the long-term future of the St. Lawrence operations. The company claimed that it was considering organizational and technological changes to help make the St. Lawrence mines more competitive with those elsewhere that could provide cheaper fluorspar.[29] Newfluor concluded that the mines could be kept open if the company built a more advanced crushing and flotation mill, which might require "some measure of involvement" from the federal and provincial governments" (*Evening Telegram* June 15, 1977). Many at St. Lawrence believed that bad news was imminent (*Evening Telegram* June 15, 1977). The union president suggested that the decision to shut down the mines had already been made and that the company was simply "prolonging the agony under the guise of more studies." However, he remained unsure of whether the company was serious about the prospect of shutting down or attempting some kind of "bluff" (*Daily News* June 20, 1977).

It was not a bluff. In July 1977, Newfluor announced that it was closing the St. Lawrence mines effective February 1978.[30] The news was met by bitterness and criticism among many at St. Lawrence. A miner approached by a journalist for a comment on the announcement responded angrily, "Why the hell should I talk to the media? When did you ever care that we existed? Soon no one need care because we won't exist. Our mine will be gone and all we'll have a monument is our cemetery" (*Evening Telegram* September 3, 1977). One woman claimed that the provincial government should have "fired broadsides into the conglomerate" and "shamed the company into reconsideration of its cruel intention." She also attacked the CNTU for being "strangely silent during the past few months" (*Southern Post* July 28, 1977). This remark had some merit: the CNTU seems to have withdrawn from involvement once the announcement was made. The depth of this woman's bitterness is evident in her claim that the sight of a roll of Alcan foil on the shelf of the supermarket sickens me. The commercial on the screen of the television set, urging me to buy Alcan siding, nauseates me…. Equally nauseating are the noises being made at the government level concerning the reduction of the economic impact on this tiny Newfoundland community.

The reaction among others was a mixture of resentment and relief, particularly on the part of women, some of whom "greeted the news with joy, but were sad to think it hadn't happened before a lot of their husbands died from radiation" (*Southern Post* July 28, 1977). One woman was quoted as saying, "too bad they didn't leave 20 years ago" (*Evening Telegram* July 25, 1977).

The company and the government also came under attack from several other quarters. The district's provincial representative criticized the company for abandoning its St. Lawrence workers to "exploit the slave labour of Mexico" (*Evening Telegram* July 25, 1977). Others challenged Alcan to make public the findings of its recent feasibility study to prove that St. Lawrence was not still a viable operation. The provincial government was criticized for not having done more to prevent the closure and the federal government for not introducing protective tariffs (*Southern Post* July 25, 1977).

One worker stated: "The reason they left here was people were kicking up quite a bit, but they were only kicking up for their right. They went to Mexico, they didn't want the hassle."[31] Another who was also put out of work by the closure suggested the company left because of "so many people dying" and the availability of cheaper ore on the world market.[32] Herbert Slaney had been involved in devising a plan, at the request of Alcan, to bring production costs down to a level where mining would be feasible. He stated that Alcan rejected the plan because it was never sincere in wanting it to succeed. What the company was ultimately after, Herbert Slaney suggested, was an uninterrupted supply of fluorspar, which it no longer believed it could get at St. Lawrence, and "They had established the alternative source before and wanted out at any cost."[33]

A look at developments over the decade or so prior to the closure seems to support this view. Shipments of fluorspar into Canada from Mexican suppliers had increased substantially during the 1960s, more than doubling in the period from 1963 to 1970 (Canada, Department of Mines and Technical Surveys 1970, 232). In 1968, Alcan began acquiring fluorspar from Mexico to meet increased demand at its Quebec smelters. Significantly, during periods of labour unrest at St. Lawrence, Alcan's imports from Mexico increased sharply (United States Bureau of Mines 1968, 218). In deciding to shut down the St. Lawrence mines, it seems Alcan was simply making more permanent a practice that had emerged over the previous decade, when it turned to foreign sources to make up for shortfalls in supply.

Dying With Money or Living Without: The Post-Newfluor Years

By the time Alcan locked its mine gates for the last time in 1978, seventy-eight miners had died from lung cancer — in addition to those who had died from other cancers or from silicosis and other pulmonary diseases. An additional 120 workers from the pre-1960 period alone were still at risk (Couves and Wright 1977, 495–98). By 1988, the official number of lung cancer deaths was 116, and seventy-two others had died from other types of cancer (including twenty-two from stomach cancer). Silicosis, pneumoconiosis, and other obstructive lung diseases had claimed twenty-eight others (Morrison 1988, 45, 52).

Closure of the Newfluor mines forced many to leave St. Lawrence for employment elsewhere. St. Lawrence was one of the very few communities in the province to experience a population decrease during the period 1978 to 1981 (Statistics Canada 1981). In 1979, a fish processing plant was established there with the assistance of the provincial government. The plant provided jobs for up to 200 people at times, but seldom on a stable, year-round basis (*Evening Telegram* February 28, 1983).

In 1983, with the fish plant all but shut down, a British-based company known as Minworth took advantage of generous provincial tax breaks and other concessions to establish a subsidiary called St. Lawrence Fluorspar and begin reactivating a mine at Blue Beach. Four hundred men signed up for the hundred jobs available. One veteran miner depicted in stark terms the dilemma many faced: "It's just as well to die with money as live without" (Story 1987, 186).

The Minworth operation is invariably described as haphazard and poorly managed. The federal government provided funding for construction of a mill and other surface works while the company was to develop the mine itself. The initial plan was to develop the mine fully before beginning to extract ore, but the company moved into mining as soon as the mill was completed. One of the results of this was that the development of the mine soon outpaced the infrastructure in such areas as ventilation. Radiation was monitored regularly by a company monitor and periodically by a government monitor, and high readings were not uncommon.[34]

There were also serious safety concerns. For example, a common procedure for safeguarding against falling rock is installing "rockbolts," which expand when inserted to tighten rock on mine ceilings, along with steel mesh to catch any rock that does fall. At the Minworth operation, rockbolts were in short supply, and workers had to remove chainlink fence from around the surface works to use as ceiling screen. Such conditions were made more dangerous by the high proportion of inexperienced workers. Many veteran miners had moved away, died, or were too old or ill to work. Others were prohibited from working underground because of their previous exposure.[35]

Initially there was no union, but hazards soon convinced workers to form one, Local 9220 of the United Steelworkers of America. However, problems with health and safety and the lack of planning continued to plague the operation. What union president Jerome Slaney called "the straw that broke the camel's back" came in February 1990. A worker was crushed to death by a slab of rock that had been hanging for two days from the ceiling of the stope he had been ordered into. According to the union president, this event "poisoned" an already negative atmosphere and the operation "never really got back on track."[36]

Around the same time as that fatality, five miners were exposed to high radiation, reportedly because a component of the ventilation system had frozen and readings had not been done. Radiation and Medical Services of the Canadian Atomic Control Board gave its assurance that such a short exposure posed no health risk, but that did little to reduce tensions. Jerome Slaney argued that "if the company would follow the rules and regulations set out in the OHS Act [the Occupational Health and Safety Act passed in 1978] and the safety policies and procedures put forward by management and the bargaining unit, there would be no problems or conflict between management and the union in regards to health and safety" (*Southern Gazette* February 10, 1990). The incident did prompt the Occupational Health and Safety Division of the Newfoundland Department of Labour to consider laying charges against the company (*Southern Gazette* February 17, 1990). However, before any decision had been made in that regard the company declared bankruptcy and soon left town.

There is no evidence at this point of any health effects from the Minworth operation, but should any of those who worked at Minworth develop an industrial disease, they may have a difficult time obtaining compensation benefits. In 1983 the Workers' Compensation Act was amended, likely as part of the concessions granted to Minworth, so that many of the provisions regarding St. Lawrence miners applied only to those who were employed in mining before January 1, 1984.

Meanwhile, effects from the earlier years continued to be felt long after the Newfluor mine was shut down. By 1990, there were 142 dead from lung cancer alone among those who had worked underground (Morrison and Villeneuve 2005, 68). Workers' compensation also continued to be an issue. A 1991 provincial government survey found that many compensation recipients were still living in substandard housing on inadequate incomes. Benefits paid out under the Special Fund had not increased since its introduction in 1971. Widows and disabled miners continued to be frustrated by what they experienced as an overly bureaucratic and arbitrary compensation system. In many cases, women had their compensation benefits terminated upon their husband's death for various technical reasons — reasons they either disagreed with or did not understand (Town Council of St. Lawrence 1996). In addition, a legislative change made in conjunction with limiting coverage to pre-1983 claims also turned out to have a detrimental effect on former workers and dependents seeking compensation. This was the elimination of coverage for surface workers by removing reference to the "handling" of fluorspar that had been introduced in 1973. Since then several claims related to former surface workers have been denied on this basis, though there appears to be no rational grounds for the change.

By 2001, the official death toll from lung cancer among underground miners was 191. The incidence of lung cancer among miners was of course still considerably higher than normal, but so was the incidence of both stomach and bladder cancer. Twenty-eight miners had died from stomach cancer and eleven from bladder cancer to that point. Sixty-four others were known to have died from silicosis and other respiratory diseases. Significantly, twenty-eight of the lung cancer deaths were among those who had started work after 1960. In many cases considerable time had elapsed between last exposure and death from lung cancer: in about forty cases, the lag time had been twenty-five to thirty-four years, while in twenty-four others it had been thirty-five years or more. (Morrison and Villeneuve 2005, 68). In addition, in a 2006 submission to a committee reviewing the workers' compensation legislation the St. Lawrence Town Council noted what it claims to be a higher than average incidence of heart and circulatory illnesses among former miners as well as the hardship created by recent policy changes like the elimination of Permanent Functional Impairment benefits for cancer victims, partly on the grounds that certain cancers may ultimately be curable (Town Council of St. Lawrence 1996, 14–21).

For many of the 1,000 or so people who live in St. Lawrence today, it is a tough place to find steady employment. The official employment rate is around 40 percent, which is low even by the standards that prevail in much of the province. A moratorium imposed on the cod fishery in 1992 further depressed an already marginal economy and led to heavy out-migration from communities like St. Lawrence. Small wonder, therefore, that some still hope for the mines to re-open. Others are dreading a repeat of the tragic nightmare. Still others, no doubt, are pondering whether there is some tolerable mix of the two. The ambivalence is evident in the words of a former miner: "I hope it never opens again… although it could be a good thing… I suppose."[37]

Notes

1. W.R. Callahan, Minister of Mines, Agriculture and Resources, to Smallwood, 19 February 1970, Coll 075, File 3.27.037, CNSA.
2. Leo Slaney, SLWPU, to W.J. Keough, Minister of Labour, 28 May 1970, MM.

3. Leo Slaney, SLWPU, to W.J. Keough, Minister of Labour, 28 May 1970, MM.
4. Stephen A. Neary, Minister of Public Welfare, to Leo Slaney, SLWPU, 31 March 1970, MM.
5. Fintan Aylward to Smallwood, 30 November 1970, Coll 075, File 3.27.037, CNSA.
6. SLWPU, Press Release, 5 February 1971, MM.
7. SLWPU, Press Release, 5 February 1971, MM.
8. St. Lawrence Town Council to Smallwood, 26 May 1971, and Smallwood to St. Lawrence Town Council, 1 June 1971, Coll 075, File 3.27.037, CNSA.
9. J.W. Cameron, Aluminum Company of Canada, to Smallwood, 28 July 1971, Coll 075, File 3.27.037, CNSA.
10. St. Lawrence Special Fund, Coll 075, File 3.21.048, CNSA.
11. M.E. Gooding, Manager, Newfluor Works, to Fred Gover, Deputy Minister of Mines, 14 January 1972, MM.
12. Reports of Radiation Readings, 1972; and David Rex to Chief Inspector of Mines (cc: Newfluor Works and SLWPU), 28 September 1972, MM.
13. George Doyle, President, SLWPU to T. Alex Hickman, Minister of Justice, 27 November 1972, MM.
14. Brief in Support of Certain Proposed Changes in the Workmen's Compensation Act Respectfully Submitted to Government of Newfoundland and Labrador by the St. Lawrence Workers' Protective Union, 7 February 1973, 6–7, MM.
15. Report of Safety Inspection, Tarefare Mine, 17 May 1974, MM; Rene Fowler, Senior Radiation Monitor, Newfluor Works, to R.R. March, Chief Inspector of Mines, 23 August 1974, MM; David Rex, Radiation Monitoring Technician, to R.R. March, 25 October 1974, MM.; and A.B. Dory, Chief Mine Engineer, Newfluor Works, to R.R. March, 4 November 1974, MM.
16. Statement for the Press by Gerard Gingras, President of the Aluminum Branch of the Federation of Mines, Metallurgy and Chemical Products (CNTU), 4 November 1974, MM.
17. Statement by Mr. J.N. Gillis, Works Manager of Alcan Newfluor Works, 7 June 1975, MM.
18. Interview with Richard Loder, October 15, 2000.
19. Interview with Herbert Slaney, October 13, 2000.
20. Interview with Richard Loder, October 15, 2000.
21. Interview with Jerome Spearns, November 28, 1998.
22. Interview with Herbert Slaney, October 13, 2000.
23. Occupational Health and Safety (with Particular Reference to Mining Operations), Status of Briefs Submitted, 1975, MM.
24. Minutes of General Membership Meeting, 18 December 1975, MM.
25. Letter from J.N. Gillis, Newfluor Manager, to members of the SLWPU, 19 December 1975, MM.
26. T.A. Blanchard, Deputy Minister of Manpower and Industrial Relations, to Michael Slaney, President, SLWPU (CNTU), 5 February 1976, MM.
27. D.J. Mitchell, Update on Alcan Smelters, 4 June 1976. MM.
28. Union List, December 1976, MM.
29. D.J. Mitchell, Newfluor, to M. Slaney, SLWPU, 27 February 1977, MM.
30. Press Release: Alcan to Close Fluorspar Mines in Newfoundland, 22 July 1977,

MM.

31. Interview with Jerome Spearns, 28 November 1998.
32. Interview with Richard Loder, 15 October 2000.
33. Interview with Herbert Slaney, 13 October 2000.
34. Interview with Jerome Slaney, 27 January 2006.
35. Interview with Jerome Spearns, 28 November 1998.
36. Interview with Jerome Slaney, 27 January 2006.
37. Interview with Jerome Spearns, 28 November 1998.

Chapter 7

CONCLUSION

When Walter Seibert sailed into St. Lawrence in the early 1930s with his boatload of rundown equipment, he found a people willing to undergo any sacrifice for the promise of paying jobs. Over the next several years, the St. Lawrence Corporation took full advantage of this desperation and the lack of alternatives. It was aided in this by the position the government of the day maintained towards occupational health and safety, public relief, and job creation, all issues intertwined with the dependence on any foreign developer that would help relieve pressure on the state, regardless of the conditions of employment. Even under such daunting circumstances, workers did not passively accept the "jobs or health" bargain, and rebelled through the limited channels available.

It was not a shift in policy or of attitudes on the part of employers or the government but a changing economic and industrial climate that eventually allowed workers to take effective action on having their concerns addressed. The entry of a second employer and the general economic improvement that accompanied the war gave workers bargaining power they had never had before, power reflected in union formation and the first mass walkout in 1940. Once again, however, the state refused to take action on workers' explicit health concerns and preserved the status quo, much to the benefit of the St. Lawrence Corporation.

The disputes of 1941 were yet another instance, this time more sustained and widespread, of workers attempting despite constraints to better their situation. The events of 1941 and the outcome of the Trade Dispute Board investigation are instructive in a number of other ways. Ultimately, this opportunity to curtail the impending tragedy was overlooked in favour of meeting market demands. Nevertheless, this situation demonstrated again that economic and industry circumstances, including a pressing demand for the mines' product, could enable workers to take action and prompt the government and employer to accede somewhat to their demands. Throughout the labour disputes and lobbying efforts of 1941, however, the employer insisted that occupational health was covered under legislation, and both the government and the employer persisted in pushing health hazards off the labour relations agenda. These actions thus underscore why conflict associated with health hazards often takes place outside the formal labour relations context. The refusal to act on workers' concerns over health hazards highlights the pattern of externalization that had been established, under which employers were able to offload the health costs of production onto workers, their families, and eventually the state.

The more difficult question suggested by developments during the early years of the war is why workers continued to tolerate such conditions, given the marked improvement in the economic situation and the possibility of finding employment elsewhere. Here, social and cultural considerations enter the picture. The vast majority of these men and their families had ties to the community that went back well over a century, even two. In this sense, St. Lawrence was unlike most other mining towns, which are established in conjunction with the industry, and this fact likely shaped the nature, extent, and ultimately recognition of the tragedy. Workers with such long and deep ties to the community and the area — even if they had the skills and other resources to pursue employment elsewhere — found it no simple matter to simply up and leave. Instead, workers persisted in their efforts to change the situation. Moreover, they might have done so to a greater extent had the industry downturn of the later war years not swung the pendulum the other way and stifled the possibility of protest.

By the early 1950s, it was increasingly apparent that miners were being sickened and killed by their work, though the exact picture was blurred by factors like the co-existence of multiple diseases. The union's affiliation with the AFL-CIO during this period appears to have decreased the attention paid to the issue of health hazards, perhaps because it was more difficult to pursue such a specific issue within this larger bureaucratic structure. The situation was not clarified by employers like the St. Lawrence Corporation, which rejected claims that workers were being affected by an industrial disease, or by the newly formed provincial government, which refused to take measures to assess the true extent of the problem for fear of the effect on employment and the industry. Fixated on creating and maintaining employment and on resource development, the government did little to address the cause of the problem. Its failure to enforce health and safety provisions is indicated by the discrepancy between government inspection reports and testimony given by miners, and the 1957 dust study revealed that neither the government nor the employers fulfilled their obligations.

The late 1950s and early 1960s brought evidence of an even deadlier menace in the form of radiation, which was now understood to be linked to rampant cancer among the workforce. The reaction of the various parties to these findings was also significant. Having reverted to independent status and lacking even a strike fund, workers walked off the job. Several did not return, indicating that for some, the "wages for health" bargain had become unacceptable. Once again, both employers and the government were less than zealous in their efforts to determine the extent of the problem. The St. Lawrence Corporation was particularly unhelpful, continuing to dispute the existence of industrial disease in the face of overwhelming evidence. The handling of cancer cases under workers' compensation also highlights the continuing externalization of costs, as an arrangement was made whereby Newfluor would be all but absolved of costs associated with cancer claims, while the St. Lawrence Corporation simply walked away from the problem, leaving workers and their families to bear the costs.

Through the first half of the 1960s, the union continued to complain of health hazards and to demand better protective measures. However, while health and safety became a stronger theme in labour negotiations and collective agreements, especially after affiliation with the CNTU, the main channels of protest continued to be lobbying the government and unsanctioned actions like wildcat strikes. The government and the remaining company, Newfluor, focused during this period on containing conflict and convincing workers that the health hazard was under control. However, matters came to a head in 1965, when Rennie Slaney's submission to the Workers' Compensation Review Committee and the Committee's report to government forced more decisive action in the form of the Royal Commission.

The Rennie Slaney submission and other events surrounding the appointment of the Royal Commission are significant in a number of respects. First, the fact that Rennie Slaney was able to record illnesses and deaths as he did points to another distinct feature of the St. Lawrence situation. Unlike the case with many resource towns, most of the St. Lawrence workforce was drawn from the community, and many workers stayed after they had become ill and left their jobs, a crucial factor that made it possible to track the incidence of disease. Thus, whereas the co-existence of multiple ailments and a lack of cooperation from employers and the government had inhibited the ability to determine the true nature and extent of the problem, these factors were offset by others, such as the relative lack of workforce migration. The ability to track the health impacts of the workplace in the case of St. Lawrence highlights special challenges of doing so in situations where the workforce is more transitory, as happens with the recent trend towards fly-in operations.

On a related theme, the Slaney submission and subsequent events threw into sharp relief the growing polarization between the minimalist and maximalist positions, a polarization generated by earlier developments like the refusal to cover claims originating before 1951 or claims for illnesses other than lung cancer and silicosis. The Rennie Slaney submission and the response to it also highlight the danger in relying on workers' compensation statistics as a source of information on the incidence of industrial disease.

Developments immediately before and after the Royal Commission was established also increased the role of public relations and media attention. The government insisted that the media was exaggerating the problem, for

example, while the employer complained that coverage was overly negative and tried to present a brighter picture of the situation. The union and
others in the community, including activists and ailing miners, continued to
complain of workplace hazards and their toll, but now with far more media
and public attention. Response to the triple fatality in September 1967,
underscored the fact that this kind of dramatic occurrence captures media
and public attention far more than the slow attrition from industrial disease.
Indeed, the Royal Commission itself was viewed by some as an important
public relations forum and an opportunity to cast the situation in a particular
light.

In addition, events during the mid-1960s highlight the complex process of
defining the nature and extent of this disaster. Up to this point a wide range
of elements had played a role in this process: insufficient medical facilities, a
lack of clarity about the connection between working conditions and illnesses,
economic considerations that made the government reluctant to investigate
and expose the true nature of the problem, a lack of cooperation on the
part of employers, the nature of the community and the labour force, and
the application of the workers' compensation system. From the mid-1960s
onward, the media would be added to these factors, which ranged beyond
strictly medical or scientific.

Increasing public awareness of health hazards in the mines and the toll
they had taken also contributed to the company's growing concern over
the labour supply. Increasing reluctance by those both in and outside the
St. Lawrence area to work in the mines, combined with the loss of many
experienced workers through disease, highlighted the failure to preserve the
health of the workforce and to convince workers and others that the health
hazards had been dealt with.

While the Royal Commission did a commendable job in conducting a
thorough investigation and making some significant recommendations, the
government's initial reaction did little to address the problems identified or
to quell the tide of bitterness and hostility growing in the workplace and the
community. In fact, by maintaining the status quo in such areas as which
cases would qualify for compensation, the government's response appears
to have fuelled antagonism and contributed to unrest spilling over into the
community. This was evident during the labour dispute of 1971, when
women in the community joined the striking miners. This dispute, which
was officially about wages, also demonstrated how grievances over health
hazards and disease had permeated the labour relations environment, even
in contexts where they were not the specific issues at stake.

For the government's part, its actions during the early 1970s consisted
largely of instituting in a piecemeal fashion many of the Royal Commission's
recommendations, usually to bring about a temporary truce in the hostilities.

This included establishing the Special Fund, which represented yet another instance of the employer externalizing the costs of disease by shifting it onto the government and ultimately taxpayers. The gradual extension of compensation coverage through amendments to the legislation during the early 1970s was undertaken within the continuing minimalist-maximalist debate, and in some cases demonstrates how the official recognition of diseases as work-related can result from labour or public protest and from purely political motivations.

The 1971 dispute also marked the launch of the CNTU's campaign to make the St. Lawrence situation a forum for its broader political agenda. This program became increasingly radical over subsequent years, peaking in the strike and protests of 1975, which the CNTU repeatedly used as a platform to attack a range of targets, from the federal government to corporate Quebec, and to advocate for Quebec independence. Much of this rhetoric resonated with the workforce, particularly younger workers, and further intensified the bitterness and hostility. Ultimately, however, much of it had little to do with the issues at stake in St. Lawrence.

Events in 1975 also highlighted once again how the legacy of disease and death, lingering grievances over exposure to health hazards, and ongoing condemnation of the workers' compensation system continued to permeate the atmosphere and to erase the boundaries between workplace, home, and community. This was evident in the mass, sustained actions of the women protestors and in observations such as that made by the mine manager, that negotiating about matters like wages was impossible in an environment dominated by "an emotional feeling of bitterness."

The company's decision to close the Newfluor operation in 1977 appears to have been based largely on its desire to maintain an uninterrupted supply of fluorspar and the ability to acquire that elsewhere. Interruptions in supply had been caused by the unrest that marked the 1970s, unrest fuelled by the mistrust and hostility that had built up over the years and by the actions of the CNTU. It remains an open question whether industry closure was an appropriate price for workers and others to pay for taking the actions they did. Clearly there were different opinions on that matter.

The situation at St. Lawrence today underscores the fact that while development brings benefits, it also comes with costs. This should include the cost of protecting workers' health. Where those responsible — employers and governments — fail to bear that cost, someone, sometime, will bear the cost of failing to protect workers' health. Too often that turns out to be workers, families and communities. At St. Lawrence, the benefits are long gone, but the costs still linger.

REFERENCES

Secondary Sources

I. Books and Articles

Alexander, David. 1974. "Development and Dependence in Newfoundland, 1880–1970." *Acadiensis* 4, 1.

_____. 1976a. "Newfoundland's Traditional Economy and Development to 1934." *Acadiensis* 5, 2.

_____. 1976b. "The Collapse of the Saltfish Trade and Newfoundland's Integration into the North American Economy." *Canadian Historical Association Papers*. 11, 5.

_____. 1978. "Economic Growth in the Atlantic Region, 1880 to 1940." *Acadiensis* 8, 1.

Anon. 1904. "The Water Drill as a Preventive of Miners' Phthisis." *Iron Age* 74 (August).

Antler, Steven. 1979. "The Capitalist Underdevelopment of Nineteenth Century Newfoundland." In Robert J. Brym and R. James Sacouman (eds.), *Underdevelopment and Social Movements in Atlantic Canada*. Toronto: New Hogtown Press.

Ashford, N. 1976. *Crisis in the Workplace: Occupational Disease and Injury*. Cambridge: MIT Press.

Aylward, Fintan. 1969. *Report of the Royal Commission on Radiation, Compensation, and Safety at the Fluorspar Mines, St. Lawrence, Newfoundland*. St. John's, NL: Office of the Queen's Printer.

Bacow, Lawrence. 1981. *Bargaining for Job Safety and Health*. Cambridge: MIT Press.

Baldwin, Doug. 1977. "A Study in Social Control: The Life of the Silver Miner in Northern Ontario." *Labour/Le Travailleur* 2.

Bartlett, L.S., et al. 1964. "Lung Cancer in a Fluorspar Mining Community: Prevalence of Respiratory Symptoms and Disability." *British Journal of Industrial Medicine* 21.

Bartrip, P.W.J., and S.B. Burman. 1983. *The Wounded Soldiers of Industry: Industrial Compensation Policy, 1833–1897*. Oxford: Clarendon.

Bartrip, Peter. 2006. *Beyond the Factory Gates: Asbestos and Health in Twentieth Century America*. New York: Continuum.

Bayer, Ronald (ed.). 1988. *The Health and Safety of Workers: The Politics of Professional Responsibility*. New York: Oxford University Press.

Beaumont, P.B. 1983. *Safety at Work and the Unions*. London: Croom Helm.

Bercuson, David Jay. 1978. "Tragedy at Bellevue: Anatomy of a Mine Disaster." *Labour/Le Travailleur* 3.

Black Rose Books Editorial Collective. 1975. *Quebec Labour: The Confederation of National Trade Unions Yesterday and Today*. Montreal: Black Rose Books.

Brown, Cassie. 1979. *Standing into Danger: a Dramatic Story of Shipwreck and Rescue*. Garden City, NY: Doubleday.

Brubaker, Sterling. 1967. *Trends in the World Aluminum Industry*. Baltimore: Johns Hopkins Press.

Bryder, Linda. 1985. "Tuberculosis, Silicosis, and the Slate Industry in North Wales, 1927–1939." In Paul Weindling (ed.), *The Social History of Occupational Health*. London: Croom Helm.

Burke, Gill. 1985. "Disease, Labour Migration and Technological Change: The Case of the Cornish Miners." In Paul Weindling (ed.), *The Social History of Occupational Health*. London: Croom Helm.

Campbell, Duncan C. 1985. *Mission Mondiale: Histoire d'Alcan*, Volume III. Toronto: Ontario Publishing Company.

Canada, Department of Mines and Technical Surveys. 1970. *Canadian Mineral Industry*. Ottawa: Office of the Queen's Printer.

Caulfield, Catherine. 1989. *Multiple Exposures: Chronicles of the Radiation Age*. New York: Harper and Row.

Clement, Wallace. 1981. *Hard Rock Mining: Industrial Relations and Technological Changes at INCO*. Toronto: McClelland and Stewart.

Collis, Edgar L., and Major Greenwood. 1977. *The Health of the Industrial Worker*. New York: Arno Press.

Confédération des syndicats nationaux. 1978. *Histoire du movement ouvier au Québec*. Montréal: Confédération des syndicats nationaux.

Coté, Luc. 1990. *Les enjeux du travail a L'Alcan, 1901–1951*. Hull: Editions Asticou.

Couves, Cecil M., and Earle S. Wright. 1977. "Radiation Induced Carcinoma of the Lung: The St. Lawrence Tragedy." *Journal of Thoracic and Cardiovascular Surgery* 74, 4 (October).

Cunningham, Simon. 1981. *The Copper Industry in Zambia: Foreign Mining Companies in a Developing Country*. New York: Praeger.

Daniel, Philip. 1979. *Africanisation, Nationalisation, and Inequality: Mining, Labour and the Copperbelt in Zambian Development*. Cambridge: Cambridge University Press.

David, Roger. 1976. *Blood on the Coal: The Story of the Springhill Mining Disasters*. Hantsport, NS: Lancelot Press.

de Villiers, A.J. 1966. "Cancer of the Lung in a Group of Fluorspar Miners." *Proceedings of the Sixth Canadian Cancer Research Conference, Honey Harbour, Ontario, 1964*.

de Villiers, A.J., and J.P. Windish. 1964. "Lung Cancer in a Fluorspar Mining Community: Radiation, Dust and Mortality Experience." *British Journal of Industrial Medicine* 21.

Derickson, Alan. 1988a. "Industrial Refugees: The Migration of Silicotics from the Mines of North America and South Africa in the Early 20th Century. *Labor History* 29, 1.

_____.1988b. *Workers' Health, Workers' Democracy: The Western Miners' Struggle, 1891–1925*. Ithaca: Cornell University Press.

_____. 1998a. *Black Lung: Anatomy of a Public Health Disaster*. Ithaca: Cornell University Press.

_____. 1998b. "Federal Intervention in the Joplin Silicosis Epidemic, 1911–1916." *Bulletin of the History of Medicine* 62.

Desrosiers, Richard, and Denis Héroux. 1973. *Le Travaillieur Québécois et le Syndicalisme*. Montreal: Les Presses de l'Université du Québec.

Dorman, Peter. 1996. *Markets and Morality: Economics, Dangerous Work and the Value of Human Life*. Cambridge: Cambridge University Press.

_____. 2000. *Three Preliminary Papers on the Economics of Occupational Safety and Health.* Geneva: International Labour Organization.

Farrell Edwards, Ena. 1983. *Notes Toward a History of St. Lawrence.* St. John's: Breakwater.

Fellman, Carl M. 1926. "The Mining of Fluorspar and Its Uses." *Proceedings of the Lake Superior Mining Institute* 25.

Fischer, R.P., and C.K. Howse. 1939. "Newfoundland Ships Fluorspar: Production from St. Lawrence Region, Begun in 1932, Has Increased Steadily." *Engineering and Mining Journal* 140, 7.

Garside, W.R. 1990. *British Unemployment, 1919–1939: A Study in Public Policy.* Cambridge: Cambridge University Press.

Gibbs, Graham H., and Paul Pintus. 1978. *Health and Safety in the Canadian Mining Industry.* Kingston: Queen's University Centre for Resource Studies.

Gillespie, William. 1986. *A Class Act: An Illustrated History of the Newfoundland Labour Movement.* St. John's: Creative.

Gjording, Chris N. 1991. *Conditions Not of Their Choosing: The Guaymi Indians and Mining Multinationals in Panama.* Washington: Smithsonian Institution Press.

Graebner, W. 1988. "Private Power, Private Knowledge and Public Health: Science, Engineering and Lead Poisoning, 1900–1970." In R. Bayer (ed.), *The Health and Safety of Workers: The Politics of Professional Responsibility.* New York: Oxford University Press.

Gunderson, Murray, and Katherine Swinton. 1981. *Collective Bargaining and Asbestos Dangers at the Workplace.* Toronto: Royal Commission on Matters of Health and Safety Arising from the Use of Asbestos in Ontario.

Güntzel, Ralph P. 2000. "'Rapprocher les lieux du pouvoir': The Quebec Labour Movement and Quebec Sovereigntism, 1960–2000." *Labour, Le Travail* 46 (Fall).

Gwyn, Richard. 1974. *Smallwood: The Unlikely Revolutionary.* Toronto: McClelland and Stewart.

Ham, James M. 1975. *Report of the Royal Commission on the Health and Safety of Workers in Mines.* Toronto: Office of the Queen's Printer.

Handcock, Gordon. 1994. "The Commission of Government's Land Settlement Scheme in Newfoundland." In James Hiller and Peter Neary (eds.), *Twentieth-Century Newfoundland: Explorations.* St. John's: Breakwater.

Hanson, S.D. 1974. "Estevan 1931." In Irving Abella (ed.), *On Strike: Six Key Labour Struggles in Canada, 1919–1949.* Toronto: James and Lewis.

Harris, J. 1954. "Radon Levels Found in Mines of New York State." *Archives of Industrial Hygiene and Occupational Medicine* 10 (July).

Hewitt, D. 1976. "Radiogenic Lung Cancer in Ontario Uranium Miners, 1955–1974." In James M. Ham, *Report of the Royal Commission on the Health and Safety of Workers in Mines.* Toronto: Office of the Queen's Printer.

Howley, James P., and Alexander Murray. 1881. *Geological Survey of Newfoundland.* London: Edward Stanford.

Ison, Terence. 1978. *The Dimensions of Industrial Disease.* Kingston: Industrial Relations Centre, Queen's University.

_____. 1979. *Occupational Health and Wildcat Strikes.* Kingston: Industrial Relations Centre, Queen's University.

Jacoe, P.W. 1953. "Occurrence of Radon in Non-Uranium Mines in Colorado." *Archives of Industrial Hygiene and Occupational Medicine* 8 (August).

James, Marcus. 1993. "The Struggle Against Silicosis in the Australian Mining Industry: The Role of the Commonwealth Government, 1920–1950." *Labour History* 65 (November).

Judkins, Bennett M. 1986. *We Offer Ourselves as Evidence: Toward Workers Control of Occupational Health.* New York: Greenwood Press.

Kealey, Gregory S. 1995. "The Canadian State's Attempt to Manage Class Conflict." In Gregory S. Kealey (ed.), *Workers and Canadian History.* Montreal and Kingston: McGill-Queen's University Press.

Labrador Institute of Northern Studies. 1982. *Labrador West Dust Study.* Labrador: The Institute.

Lanning, G., and M. Mueller. 1979. *Africa Undermined: A History of Mining Companies and the Underdevelopment of Africa.* Middlesex: Penguin Books.

Leyton, Elliot. 1975a. *Dying Hard: The Ravages of Industrial Carnage.* Toronto: McClelland and Stewart.

_____. 1975b. "The Bad Death." *Maclean's* 88.

Litvak, Isaiah A., and Christopher J. Maule. 1977. *Royal Commission on Corporate Concentration, Study No. 13: Alcan Aluminum Limited.* Ottawa: Carleton University.

Logan, Harold. 1948. *Trade Unions in Canada: Their Development and Functioning.* Toronto: MacMillan.

Lord Amulree. 1933. *Report of the Newfoundland Royal Commission, 1933.* London: HM Stationery Office.

Lunn, Robert, and Bryan D. Palmer. 1997. "The Big Sleep: The Malartic Mine Fire of 1947." *Labour/Le Travail* 39 (Spring).

MacDowell, Laurel S. 1978. "The Formation of the Canadian Industrial Relations System During World War Two." *Labour/Le Travailleur* 3.

MacKay, R.A. 1946. *Newfoundland: Economic, Diplomatic and Strategic Studies.* Toronto: Oxford University Press.

Markowitz, Gerald, and David Rosner. 1987. *Dying for Work: Safety and Health in the United States.* Bloomington: Indiana University Press.

Martin, Wendy. 1983. *Once Upon a Mine: Story of Pre-Confederation Mines on the Island of Newfoundland.* Montreal: Canadian Institute of Mining and Metallurgy.

Martland, Sandra. 1978. "Resisting Multinational Asbestos: The Struggle for Workplace Safety in Newfoundland." *Alternatives* 7, 4 (Autumn).

Marx, Karl. 1977. *Capital: A Critique of Political Economy*, Volume 1. Moscow: Progress Publishers.

McArthur, Jack. 1960. "Cancer Tragedy Deadly Mystery in Newfoundland." *Financial Post.* March 12.

McCormick, Christopher (ed.). 1992. *The Westray Chronicles: A Case Study in Corporate Crime.* Halifax: Fernwood Publishing.

McDonald, Ian D.H. 1987, *"To Each his Own": William Coaker and the Fishermen's Protective Union in Newfoundland Politics, 1908–1925.* J.K. Hiller (ed.). St. John's: ISER Books.

McKay, Ian. 1984. "Springhill 1958." *New Maritimes* 2 (December 1983/January 1984).

Morrison, H., and Canada, Atomic Energy Control Board. 1988. *The Mortality*

Experience of a Group of Newfoundland Fluorspar Miners Exposed to the Rn Progeny.
Ottawa: Atomic Energy Control Board.

Morrison, H., and Paul Villeneuve. 2005. "Radon-progeny Exposure and Lung
Cancer: A Mortality Study of Newfoundland Fluorspar Miners, 1950–2001."
Ottawa: Epistream Consulting, Inc..

Müller, Rainer. 1985. "A Patient in Need of Care: German Occupational Health
Statistics." In Paul Weindling (ed.), *The Social History of Occupational Health*.
London: Croom Helm.

Murray, Alexander, and James P. Howley. 1881. *Geological Survey of Newfoundland*.
London: Edward Stanford.

Neary, Peter. 1988. *Newfoundland in the North Atlantic World, 1929–1949*. Kingston-
Montreal: McGill-Queen's University Press.

Noel, S.J.R. 1971. *Politics in Newfoundland*. Toronto: University of Toronto Press.

Novek, Joel. 1992. "The Labor Process and Workplace Injuries in the Canadian
Meatpacking Industry." *Canadian Review of Sociology and Anthropology* 29: 1
(1992).

O'Faircheallaigh, Ciaran. 1984. *Mining and Development: Foreign-Financed Mines in
Australia, Ireland, Papua New Guinea and Zambia*. London: Croom Helm.

Overton, James. 1990. "Economic Crisis and the End of Democracy: Politics in
Newfoundland During the Great Depression." *Labour/Le Travail* 26 (Fall).

_____. 1994. "Self-Help, Charity, and Individual Responsibility: the Political
Economy of Social Policy in Newfoundland in the 1920s." In James Hiller
and Peter Neary (eds.), *Twentieth-Century Newfoundland: Explorations*. St. John's:
Breakwater.

_____. 1995. "Moral Education of the Poor: Adult Education and Land Settlement
Schemes in Newfoundland in the 1930s." *Newfoundland Studies* 11, 2 (Fall).

_____. 1998. "Public Relief and Social Unrest in Newfoundland in the 1930s: An
Evaluation of the Ideas of Piven and Cloward." *Canadian Journal of Sociology*
13, 1–2 (Winter-Spring).

Paehlke, Robert. 1979. "Occupational Health Policy in Canada." In William Leiss
(ed.), *Ecology Versus Politics in Canada*. Toronto: University of Toronto Press.

Parkinson, N.F. 1955. "Silicosis in Canada." *American Medical Association Archives of
Industrial Health* (July).

Piva, Michael. 1975. "The Workers' Compensation Movement in Ontario." *Ontario
History* 67.

Prowse, D.W. 1895. *A History of Newfoundland from the English, Colonial and Foreign Records*.
Belleville, ON: Mika.

Quinlan, Michael. 1999. "The Implications of Labour Market Restructuring in
Industrialized Societies for Occupational Health and Safety." *Economic and
Industrial Democracy* 20, 3.

Reasons, Charles E., et al. 1981. *Assault on the Worker: Occupational Health and Safety in
Canada*. Toronto: Butterworths.

Reeves, William. 1989. "Alexander's Conundrum Reconsidered: The American
Dimension in Newfoundland Resource Development, 1898–1910." *Newfoundland
Studies* 5, 1.

Reschenthaler, G.B. 1979. *Occupational Health and Safety in Canada: The Economics and
Three Case Studies*. Montreal: Institute for Research on Public Policy.

Robinson, Ian. 1982. *The Costs of Uncertainty: Regulating Health and Safety in the Canadian Uranium Industry.* Ottawa: Centre for Resource Studies, Institute of Intergovernmental Relations.

Robinson, James C. 1991. *Toil and Toxics: Workplace Struggles and Political Strategies for Occupational Health.* Berkeley: University of California Press.

Rosenstock, Linda, Mark R. Cullen, and Marilyn Fingerhut. 2005. "Advancing Worker Health and Safety in the Developing World." *Journal of Occupational and Environmental Medicine* 47, 2.

Rosner, David. 1992. *Deadly Dust: Silicosis and the Politics of Occupational Disease in Twentieth-Century America.* New Jersey: Princeton University Press.

Rouillard, Jacques. 1981. *Histoire de la CSN, 1921–1981.* Montreal: Boréal Express/CSN.

Ryan, Shannon. 1986. *Fish out of Water: The Newfoundland Saltfish Trade, 1814-1914.* St. John's: Breakwater.

Sanderson, H.P., and J.P. Windish. 1958. *Dust Hazards in the Mines Of Newfoundland: I. Newfoundland Fluorspar Limited, St. Lawrence, Newfoundland.* Ottawa: Laboratory Services, Occupational Health Division, Dept. of National Health and Welfare.

Sass, Robert. 1979. "The Underdevelopment of Occupational Health and Safety in Canada." In William Leiss (ed.), *Ecology Versus Politics in Canada.* Toronto: University of Toronto Press.

Seager, Allen. 1985. "Socialists and Workers: The Western Canadian Coal Miners, 1900–21." *Labour/Le Travail* 16 (Fall).

Selikoff, Irving J. 1977. *Clinical Survey of Chrysotile Asbestos Miners and Millers in Baie Verte, Newfoundland, 1976: Report to the National Institute of Environmental Health Sciences.* Baie Verte, Newfoundland: United Steelworkers of America.

Slaney, Rennie. 1975. *More Incredible than Fiction: The True Story of the Indomitable Men and Women of St. Lawrence from the Time of Settlement to 1965.* Montreal: La Confédération des Syndicats Nationeaux.

Smith, Barbara Ellen. 1987. *Digging Our Own Graves: Coalminers and the Struggle over Black Lung Disease.* Philadelphia: Temple University Press.

Smith, Doug. 2000. *Consulted to Death.* Winnipeg: Arbeiter Ring.

Statistics Canada. 1981. *Selected Population, Dwelling, Household and Census Family Characteristics.* Ottawa: Statistics Canada.

Storey, Robert, and Wayne Lewchuk. 2000. "From Dust to Dust: Asbestos and the Struggle for Worker Health and Safety at Bendix Automotive." *Labour/Le Travail* 45.

Story, Alan. 1987. "Old Wounds: Reopening the Mines of St. Lawrence." In Gary Burrill and Ian McKay (eds.), *People, Resources, and Power: Critical Perspectives on Underdevelopment and Primary Industries in Atlantic Canada.* Fredericton: Acadiensis Press.

Struthers, James. 1983. *No Fault of Their Own: Unemployment and the Canadian Welfare State, 1914–1941.* Toronto: University of Toronto Press.

Summers, Valerie. 1994. *Regime Change in a Resource Economy: The Politics of Underdevelopment in Newfoundland Since 1825.* St. John's: Breakwater.

Suschnigg, P. 1989. "Economic Conditions and Industrial Fatalities in Canada, 1928–81." *Sociology and Social Research* 74 (October).

Sutherland, Dufferin. 1992. "Newfoundland Loggers Respond to the Great Depression." *Labour/Le Travail* 29 (Spring).

Taft, Philip. 1959. *The A.F. of L. from the Death of Gompers to the Merger.* New York: Harper and Brothers.

Tataryn, Lloyd. 1979. *Dying for a Living.* Ottawa: Deneau and Greenberg.

Thompkins, R.W. 1944. "Radioactivity and Lung Cancer: A Critical Review of Lung Cancer in the Miners of Schneeberg and Joachimsthal." *Journal of the National Cancer Institute* 5.

Trudeau, Pierre Elliott. 1974. *The Asbestos Strike.* Toronto: James Lewis and Samuel.

Tucker, Eric. 1990. *Administering Danger in the Workplace: The Law and Politics of Occupational Health and Safety Regulation in Ontario.* Toronto: University of Toronto Press.

_____. 2006. "Introduction: The Politics of Recognition and Response. In Eric Tucker (ed.), *Working Disasters: The Politics of Recognition and Response.* Amityville, New York: Baywood Publishing Company.

United States Bureau of Mines. 1940. *Minerals Yearbook* Washington: Bureau of Mines.

_____. 1958. *Minerals Yearbook.* Washington: Bureau of Mines.

_____. 1968. *Minerals Yearbook.* Washington: Bureau of Mines.

Wallace, Michael. 1987. "Dying for Coal: The Struggle for Health and Safety Conditions in American Coal Mining, 1930–82." *Social Forces* 66, 2.

Webster, I. 1972. "The Pathology of Silicosis." In John. M. Rogan (ed.), *Medicine in the Mining Industries.* London: William Heinemann Medical Books.

Wedeen, Richard P. 1984. *Poison in the Pot: The Legacy of Lead.* Carbondale: Southern Illinois University Press, 1984.

Weindling, Paul. 1985. "Linking Self Help and Medical Science: The Social History of Occupational Health." In Paul Weindling (ed.), *The Social History of Occupational Health.* London: Croom Helm.

Whiteside, Noel. 1991. *Bad Times: Unemployment in British Social and Political History.* London: Faber and Faber.

Windish, J.P. 1960. *Health Hazards In The Mines Of Newfoundland: III. Radiation Levels In The Workings Of Newfoundland Fluorspar Limited, St. Lawrence, Newfoundland.* Ottawa: Department of National Health and Welfare.

Zieger, Robert H. 1977. *Madison's Battery Workers, 1934–52: A History of Federal Labour Union 1958.* Ithaca: Cornell University Press.

II. Newspapers

Daily News. February 12, 1912.

Daily News. November 23, 1929.

Daily News. March 2, 1960.

Daily News. March 18, 1960. "Radiation Picture at St. Lawrence Overemphasized Says Wiseman."

Daily News. March 11, 1960. "50 Men Quit in Fluorspar Mine."

Daily News. May 8, 1960. "Radiation Levels Safe in St. Lawrence Mines."

Daily News. October 25, 1960. "Strike by Miners at St. Lawrence."

Daily News. June 4, 1977. "Alcan Will Decide Mine's Future in June."

Daily News. June 20, 1977. "St. Lawrence's Future? Union Head Pessimistic."

Evening Telegram. February 1, 1940.

Evening Telegram. January 5, 1940.

Evening Telegram. November 7, 1941. "Fluorspar Miners Strike for More Pay."

Evening Telegram. December 6, 1941

Evening Telegram. May 20, 1949.

Evening Telegram. June 6, 1957. "Markets Lost, Fluorspar Mine Announces Shutdown."

Evening Telegram. June 8, 1957. "Government Moves to Re-open Mines Again."

Evening Telegram. March 2, 1960. "Government Officials Meet to Discuss Radiation Hazard in Fluorspar Mines."

Evening Telegram. March 2, 1960. "Miners Get More Cancer."

Evening Telegram. March 3, 1960. "Miners 'Wait and See' as Cancer Cause Checked."

Evening Telegram. March 11, 1960. "Miners Back Request as Walkout Endorsed."

Evening Telegram. March 18, 1960. "Fluorspar Mines OK, Asks End to Walkout."

Evening Telegram. March 24, 1960. "Miners Stay Out, Seek Jobless Aid."

Evening Telegram. April 1, 1960. "Ventilation System is Installed."

Evening Telegram. April 4, 1960. "St. Lawrence Miners Go Back to Work."

Evening Telegram. April 7, 1960. "Miners Scared, Won't Go Back, Union Says Company Hiring Green Men."

Evening Telegram. April 11, 1960. "St. Lawrence Mines on 24-Hour Shift."

Evening Telegram. March 31, 1967. "Compensation Should be Paid says St. Lawrence Miner."

Evening Telegram. March 31, 1967. "Tragedy Termed National Disaster."

Evening Telegram. September 18, 1967. "Killer Mine Snuffs Out Three More Lives."

Evening Telegram. September 19, 1967. "Most Dangerous Sections of Deadly Mine Closed."

Evening Telegram. September 29, 1967. "Mine Fatalities."

Evening Telegram. April 10, 1970. "St. Lawrence Strike."

Evening Telegram. June 3, 1970. "Government Response to St. Lawrence Study Draws Fire."

Evening Telegram. April 2, 1971. "Long Time Before Benefits Come, says St. Lawrence Union President."

Evening Telegram. April 6, 1971.

Evening Telegram. April 7, 1971.

Evening Telegram. April 8, 1971.

Evening Telegram. April 11, 1971.

Evening Telegram. April 12, 1971. "Strikes Continue, Over 500 Workers Out."

Evening Telegram. April 16, 1971. "St. Lawrence Workers Vote to Strike."

Evening Telegram. April 18, 1971.

Evening Telegram. April 19, 1971. "1,000 Workers Now Off Jobs."

Evening Telegram. May 14, 1971. "New Safety Measures Planned for St. Lawrence Mines."

Evening Telegram. May 7, 1971. "Breakdown Negotiations, St. Lawrence Strike Still On."

Evening Telegram. May 6, 1971. "Month-old Strike Ends at Springdale."

Evening Telegram, May 10, 1971. "St. Lawrence Strike Could Be a Long One."

Evening Telegram. June 23, 1971. "Buchans Strike Could be a Long One."

Evening Telegram. June 30, 1971. "Drug Problem Developing in St. Lawrence."

Evening Telegram. July 6, 1971.

Evening Telegram. July 6, 1971. "The Widows of St. Lawrence: Won't Somebody Out There Help Us."

Evening Telegram. July 8, 1971. "A Miner's Fate."

Evening Telegram. July 9, 1971. "Alcan Strike Enters 13th Week, Miners Not Feeling the Pinch Yet."

Evening Telegram. August 2, 1971. "At Last, Some Help."

Evening Telegram. August 2, 1971. "Special Fund Set Up in St. Lawrence for Widows and Orphans of Miners."

Evening Telegram. September 11, 1971. "23-Week Old Strike Ends at St Lawrence."

Evening Telegram. September 30, 1971. "St. Lawrence Union Head Quits."

Evening Telegram. April 2, 1973. "900 off Jobs in Strikes."

Evening Telegram. April 2, 1973. "St. Lawrence Miners Strike."

Evening Telegram. May 2, 1973. "Workmen's Compensation Payments Increased."

Evening Telegram. May 4, 1973. "Fluorspar Miners Back on Job."

Evening Telegram. June 1, 1975. "Female Picketers Jubilant."

Evening Telegram. June 11, 1975.

Evening Telegram. June 12, 1975. "'Outside' Union Officials Charged with Leading Mine Workers Astray."

Evening Telegram. "June 12, 1975. "St. Lawrence Miners Charged with Intimidation by Violence."

Evening Telegram. June 13, 1975. "Potentially Ugly Confrontation Averted as Alcan, Union Resume Negotiations."

"*Evening Telegram*. June 14, 1975. "Mining Town Residents Await Outcome of Talks."

Evening Telegram. June 21, 1975. "New Contract Won't Settle Real Issues."

Evening Telegram. June 27, 1975. "Alcan Labour Dispute Still at Standstill."

Evening Telegram. June 29, 1975. "Women Not Afraid of Alcan. 'They're Afraid of Us'."

Evening Telegram. September 29, 1975. "Miners Still Wait for UIC Benefits."

Evening Telegram. October 22, 1975. "Union Official Blasts Alcan, Company 'Savage', 'Uncivilized'."

Evening Telegram. November 1, 1975. "No UIC Benefits for Miners in St. Lawrence."

Evening Telegram. November 10, 1975.

Evening Telegram. November 14, 1975. "Miners Get Government Assurance of Stronger Legislation on Safety."

Evening Telegram. November 14, 1975. "St. Lawrence Miners, Cabinet Meeting Today."

Evening Telegram, December 12, 1975. "Miners in St. Lawrence Prepared to Go to Prison."

Evening Telegram. December 20, 1975. "Mayor Concerned Over Rejection of Wage Offer."

Evening Telegram. February 2, 1976. "Province Not Left with Many Options."

Evening Telegram. February 7, 1976. "Alcan Miners Going Back to Work."

Evening Telegram. June 15, 1977. "No News is Bad News for Alcan Employees."

Evening Telegram. July 12, 1977.

Evening Telegram. July 25, 1977. "Alcan Will Close Down Mine at St. Lawrence."

Evening Telegram. September 3, 1977. "The Real Reason Mine is Closing."

Evening Telegram. February 28, 1983.

Montreal Star. April 7, 1960. "Radiation Led to Walkout."

Newfluor News. March 1968.

Newfluor News. September 1968.

Newfluor News. October 1968.

Newfluor News. November 1968.

Newfluor News. April 1969.

Newfluor News. May 1969.

Newfluor News. June 1969. "Security Police for Newfluor."

Newfluor News. September 1971. "Special Fund Established."

Newfluor News. June 1974

Newfluor News. December 1974. "The Art of Aluminum Foil."

Newfluor News. February 1975. "Tough Year Ahead Says Alcan President."

Newfoundland Journal of Commerce. June 6, 1957. "Will St. Lawrence Become a Ghost Town?"

Northern Miner. March 31, 1960. "St. Lawrence Corporation to Resume Output at Fluorspar Mines.

Southern Gazette. February 10, 1990. "Exposed Miners Not at Health Risk."

Southern Gazette. February 17, 1990. "Government Considering Laying Charges Against St. Lawrence Fluorspar."

Southern Post. July 25, 1977. "If Trudeau Phoned, He Says, St. Lawrence Would Not Close."

Southern Post. July 28, 1977. "What Will Save St. Lawrence?"

Southern Post. July 28, 1977. "Sixty Percent Surface Work Completed."

III. Government Publications

Newfoundland Chief Electoral Officer. 1956. *Official List of Electors, 1955*. St. John's: Office of the Queen's Printer.

Newfoundland Department of Finance. 1970. *Historical Statistics of Newfoundland and Labrador*. St. John's: Office of the Queen's Printer.

Newfoundland Department of Mines and Resources. 1954. *Annual Report for the Year Ended 31 March 1953*. St. John's: Office of the Queen's Printer.

_____. 1955. *Annual Report for the Year Ended 31 March 1954*. St. John's: Office of the Queen's Printer.

_____. 1956. *Annual Report for the Year Ended 31 March 1955*. St. John's: Office of the Queen's Printer.

_____. 1957. *Annual Report for the Year Ended 31 March 1956*. St. John's: Office of the Queen's Printer.

_____. 1961. *Annual Report for the Year Ended 31 March 1960*. St. John's: Office of the Queen's Printer.

Newfoundland Department of Mines, Agriculture and Resources. 1964. *Annual Report for the Year Ended 31 March 1963*. St. John's: Office of the Queen's Printer.

_____. 1968. *Annual Report for the Year Ended 31 March 1967*. St. John's: Office of the Queen's Printer.

Newfoundland Department of Public Health and Welfare. 1946. *Eleventh Census of Newfoundland and Labrador, 1945*. St. John's: Office of the King's Printer.

_____. 1936. *Tenth Census of Newfoundland and Labrador 1935*. St. John's: Office of the King's Printer.

Newfoundland. 1877. *Journal of the House of Assembly of Newfoundland*. St. John's: Office of the King's Printer.

_____. 1887. *Journal of the House of Assembly of Newfoundland*. St. John's: Office of the King's Printer.

_____. 1909. *Statutes of Newfoundland*. St. John's: Office of the King's Printer.

_____. 1909b. *Statutes of Newfoundland*. St. John's: Office of the King's Printer.

_____. 1941. *Report of the Tribunal in the Matter of the Strike at Buchans Mine, Newfoundland, August 1ˢᵗ to 14ᵗʰ, 1941*. St. John's: Office of the King's Printer.

_____. 1941b. *Acts of the Honourable Commission of Government of Newfoundland*. St. John's: Office of the King's Printer.

_____. 1942. *Settlement of Trade Dispute Board Appointed for the Settlement of a Dispute Between the St. Lawrence Corporation of Newfoundland and the St. Lawrence Workers' Protective Union*. St. John's: Office of the King's Printer.

_____. 1952. *Statutes of Newfoundland*. St. John's: Office of the King's Printer.

_____. September 29, 1959. *The Newfoundland Gazette*. St. John's: Office of the Queen's Printer.

_____. March 29, 1960. *The Newfoundland Gazette*. St. John's: Office of the Queen's Printer.

_____. 1961. *Statutes of Newfoundland*. St. John's: Office of the Queen's Printer

_____. March 7, 1967. *The Newfoundland Gazette*. St. John's: Office of the Queen's Printer.

_____. 1970b. *Journal of the House of Assembly of Newfoundland*. St. John's: Office of the Queen's Printer.

_____. 1972. *Statutes of Newfoundland*. St. John's: Office of the Queen's Printer.

_____. 1973. *Statutes of Newfoundland*. St. John's: Office of the Queen's Printer.

_____. 1974. *Statutes of Newfoundland*. St. John's: Office of the Queen's Printer.

_____. 1976. *Statutes of Newfoundland*. St. John's: Office of the Queen's Printer.

_____. 1979. *Report of the Royal Commission into the Cause or Causes of Three industrial Accidents Involving Death Which Occurred in January and February, 1977, within the Mines and Property of the Iron Ore Company of Canada Situated Near Labrador City*. St. John's: Office of the Queen's Printer.

Nova Scotia. 1952. *Statutes of Nova Scotia*. Halifax. Office of the King's Printer.

Ontario.1949. *Statutes of Ontario*. Toronto: Office of the King's Printer.

IV. Unpublished

Canada, Department of Finance. 1958. "Report of the Tariff Board Relative to the Investigation Ordered by the Minister of Finance Respecting Fluorspar Ottawa." Centre for Newfoundland Studies, Memorial University of Newfoundland.

Fogwill, Irving. 1950. "Report of the Workmen's Compensation Committee of Newfoundland on the Organization and Administration of a Workmen's

Compensation Board for Newfoundland." St. John's, NL: Centre for Newfoundland Studies, Memorial University of Newfoundland.

Hiley, Walter M. 1945. "Fluorspar Policies of the War Production Board and Predecessor Agencies, May 1940 to June 1945." In the possession of the author.

Kealey, Gregory S. 1986. "The History and Structure of the Newfoundland Labour Movement: Background Report Prepared for Royal Commission on Employment and Unemployment, Newfoundland and Labrador." St. John's, NL: Centre for Newfoundland Studies, Memorial University of Newfoundland.

Leyton, Elliot.1977a. "Public consciousness and public policy. Proceedings of Conference of the Canadian Ethnology Society." St. John's, NL: Centre for Newfoundland Studies, Memorial University of Newfoundland.

_____. 1977b. "The bureaucratization of anguish: The Workmen's Compensation Board in an industrial disaster." St. John's NL: Centre for Newfoundland Studies, Memorial University of Newfoundland.

Newfoundland. 1929. Report by Inspector J.H. Dee on Disaster of Night of 18th November, on the Coast from Lamaline to St. Lawrence, Inclusive. St. John's, NL: Centre for Newfoundland Studies, Memorial University of Newfoundland.

Newfoundland. 1970. Decisions of the Government on the Report of the Royal Commission Respecting Radiation, Compensation, and Safety at the Fluorspar Mines, St. Lawrence. St. John's, NL: Center for Newfoundland Studies, Memorial University of Newfoundland.

Peat, Marwick, Mitchell and Company. 1950. "Report on Application for Financial Assistance, St. Lawrence Corporation of Newfoundland, Limited, and St. Lawrence Fluorspar Inc." St. John's, NL: Centre for Newfoundland Studies, Memorial University of Newfoundland.

Town Council of St. Lawrence. 1996. "Brief by the St. Lawrence Town Council to the Statutory Review Committee of Workers' Compensation ." In the possession of the author.

Town Council of St. Lawrence. 2006. "Brief by the St. Lawrence Town Council to the Statutory Review Committee of Workers' Compensation ." In the possession of the author.

Trist, Eric L. 1968. "The Situation at Newfoundland Fluorspar Limited in relation to the St. Lawrence Community." In the possession of the author.

Winter, H.A. 1966. "Report of the Review Committee Appointed to Review, Consider, Report Upon and Make Recommendations Respecting the Workmen's Compensation Act." St. John's, NL: Centre for Newfoundland Studies, Memorial University of Newfoundland.

Primary Sources

I. Archival

Archival Collection of the Aluminum Company of Canada, Montreal.

Archival Collection of the St. Lawrence Memorial Miners' Museum, St. Lawrence, Newfoundland.

Centre for Newfoundland Studies Archive, Memorial University of Newfoundland.

Hagley Museum and Library, Wilmington, Delaware.

Memorial University of Newfoundland Folklore and Language Archive, St. John's, Newfoundland.

National Archives of Canada, Ottawa

Provincial Archives of Newfoundland and Labrador, St. John's, Newfoundland.

Records of the Dominions Office, Centre for Newfoundland Studies, Memorial University of Newfoundland, St. John's, NL.

Records of the Newfoundland and Labrador Department of Mines and Energy, St. John's, NL.

II. Interviews

Richard Clarke, Little St. Lawrence, October 26, 1997.

Richard Loder, St. Lawrence, October 15, 2000.

Adrian Slaney, St. Lawrence, February 7, 2000.

Herbert Slaney, St. Lawrence, October 13, 2000.

Jerome Spearns, Little St. Lawrence, November 28, 1998.

Jerome Slaney, St. Lawrence, January 27, 2006.